SHIFTING NARRATIVES

ANITA COMISKY AND MICHELLE BELLOIT

ISBN: 978-1-960136-62-6

Table of Contents

Introduction

In the pages that follow, we will embark on a journey together. We will explore the stories of ten extraordinary women who have walked in your shoes, felt that same sense of emptiness and longing, and dared to take the leap of faith toward self-discovery and fulfillment. These women have found their passions, discovered their purposes, and now radiate joy in a truly inspiring way. They are living proof that it is never too late to start over.

As we delve into their stories, you will find inspiration, guidance, and practical advice on how to fill the void in your life. You will learn through their stories how they identified their passions, set goals, overcame obstacles, and created a deeply meaningful and fulfilling life. What's more, you will realize that you are not alone on your journey; there is a vibrant community of women ready to support and encourage you every step of the way.

Each of the remarkable women we'll introduce you to in this book embarked on a transformative journey driven by a powerful force within them. They found the courage to break free from the shackles of the mundane, to overcome the daunting challenges that lay in their path. But what ignited this inner spark? What fueled their desire for change and fulfillment?

One common theme united them all: a deep sense of restlessness. They experienced anger, frustration, and a profound sense of powerlessness. The reasons behind these emotions were as diverse as the women themselves. Some had faced the painful aftermath of divorce, navigating the turbulent waters of legal battles and emotional turmoil. Others had realized that their once-loving marriages had devolved into mere roommate arrangements, devoid of passion and affection. Still others grappled with the weight of dysfunctional family dynamics, unable to break free.

Yet, despite the unique circumstances that led them to this point, the emotions they felt were universally relatable. These emotions became the catalyst for transformation, the driving force behind their quest for fulfillment.

Anger, when harnessed positively, can become a powerful source for change. It is the emotional response to injustice, to the recognition that something is amiss. These women channeled their anger, not into bitterness or despair, but into the fuel that ignited their desire for something better.

Frustration, too, played a pivotal role. It's that sense of being stuck in a rut, of facing the same challenges repeatedly. It's the realization that the current path isn't leading to the desired destination. Frustration can be a gift, pushing us to seek alternatives and make necessary changes.

Powerlessness, perhaps the most challenging emotion of all, often precedes significant transformation. It's the feeling that we lack control over our lives, that external forces are dictating our choices. Yet it is precisely in this moment of vulnerability that we can find the strength to reclaim our agency and rewrite our stories.

As you read through these pages, you may find yourself wondering if this book holds the inspiration and encouragement you need to move forward. Let us assure you, it most certainly does. We have delved deep into the lives of these incredible women to unearth what motivated them, what sustained them, and what ultimately led them to their destinies. Their stories are not just anecdotes but profound lessons in resilience, determination, and the unwavering belief that a better life is within reach.

We all face difficult moments in our lives when it seems like we're caught in a never-ending cycle of mediocrity, when our dreams feel distant, and our spirits wane. Sometimes, we lack the knowledge, ability, or energy to break free from these negative feelings. However, the stories we are about to share with you have the power to change that. They will light a fire within you, fueling your passion and drive to take that next step toward your goals and dreams.

During our conversations with these remarkable women, we were struck by the audacity of their choices. They had, in essence, left behind lives that were comfortable, lives that they had become accustomed to, in pursuit of something more fulfilling. As we listened to their narratives, it became abundantly clear that their decisions were far from easy. They had to confront doubts, conquer fears, and challenge societal expectations to follow their hearts and chase their dreams.

Each woman had embarked on a courageous journey of transformation, leaving behind the familiar and stepping into the unknown. They were moving from lives of complacency to lives of contentment, and we couldn't help but wonder—what was it that enabled them to make this shift? What was the driving force behind their audacious choices?

Their stories revealed a profound sense of freedom—a freedom that transcended the mere absence of constraints and limitations. It was the liberation they felt, the freedom to make choices that resonated with their true selves, and the autonomy to define life on their own terms.

No longer shackled by societal norms or obligations, this newfound freedom encouraged them to seize fresh opportunities, explore their desire within, and, most importantly, discover authentic happiness. The transformation they experienced was not just external; it was a deep, internal shift—a transformation of their soul.

In the pages that follow, we will dive deeper into these women's stories, exploring the various facets of the freedom they embraced. We will dissect the power of autonomy, the courage to defy norms, and the exhilaration of making choices aligned with one's innermost desires.

But before we do that, we encourage you to take a moment to reflect on your own life. Are there areas where you feel bound by expectations, where you sense a longing for more, a yearning for a life that truly reflects your essence?

We invite you to sit back, relax, and let these tales of perseverance and triumph inspire you. Allow them to kindle that spark within you and watch it grow into a raging inferno of motivation and success. Your journey begins now.

Section 1 Introduction - Adventurous

In life, there often comes a moment when the familiar routines and responsibilities no longer bring satisfaction. For many of the women in our stories, a feeling of disappointment seeped in gradually, showing up as a quiet dissatisfaction that clouded daily experiences and accomplishments.

There were moments when the colors seemed to fade, and the threads lost their luster. Moments when the rhythm of existence felt more like a monotonous drone than a symphony of joy. For many women, this moment arrived quietly, creeping into their consciousness like a thief in the night. They had feelings of disenchantment, a sense that the life they were living no longer resonated with their deepest desires and aspirations.

In the chapters ahead, we share the stories of women's journeys as they shift their narratives, illustrating how they transformed their lives into meaningful journeys of self-discovery and fulfillment.

The stories you will read here all share common threads and themes that resonate deeply and universally. Each woman, all over 40, found herself at a significant crossroads, feeling an urgent need to shift her narrative. They had reached a point in their lives best described as "paused". A state often precipitated by profound life changes such as divorce, the death of a loved one, or significant career upheavals. These pauses were not mere momentary lulls, but were deeply entrenched in the habit of looking back at their pasts with regret or down at their current circumstances with a sense of despair. This backward and downward focus was a substantial factor contributing to their stagnation.

However, each woman experienced a pivotal moment when she decided to shift her narrative. This shift was not just a change in their stories, but a profound transformation in how they perceived their lives. By consciously redirecting their focus from what was behind them or beneath them, they began to look forward and outward, embracing new possibilities and opportunities. This transformative shift in perspective allowed them to break free from the confines of their paused states.

In this process of rewriting their own narratives, they started to create lives imbued with light, hope, and joy. They discovered a renewed sense of purpose and passion, fostering resilience and strength. Despite facing daunting challenges, these women chose to rewrite their stories with grace and optimism. They found ways to cultivate happiness and fulfillment, proving that it's never too late to transform one's life. Their journeys are a testament to the power of narrative change, illustrating how altering one's perspective can lead to profound personal growth and a more vibrant, hopeful future.

CHAPTER 1

How to Design a Second Act

*"Selling my business marked a bittersweet victory;
it was a leap into a new chapter, leaving behind the
exhilarating chaos of entrepreneurship for the peace that comes
with knowing I had finally chosen to prioritize my well-being
over the relentless grind."*

The day I sold my business was a day of both triumph and mild regret. In my 30s and early 40s, I was living the high-octane life of a business owner. Think caffeine-fueled days, sleepless nights, and a to-do list that looked more like a novel. My business always required constant attention. The adrenaline rush of growing a lucrative business was exhilarating, but after more than a decade, the 24/7 grind left me feeling more frazzled than fulfilled. I was running on fumes, and the thrill had worn off.

One particularly grueling day, my husband and I had a heart-to-heart. We were both exhausted and craved a change. We did what any sane couple on the brink of burnout would do: we started planning our escape. We meticulously calculated how much we would need to retire comfortably. This wasn't just a number scribbled on a cocktail napkin; this was the product of years of hard work and savvy financial planning. We crunched the numbers, debated the finer points of what "enough" looked like for retirement, and finally settled on a figure that would allow us to live comfortably without having to work another day. With that magic number in mind, we slapped a sale price on the business.

We sat across from the buyer, a former customer, and named our price. When we presented our asking price to our prospective buyer and braced for negotiation, they didn't even flinch. My husband and I exchanged a glance, both of us mentally kicking ourselves for not aiming higher. But hey, hindsight is 20/20, and besides, we were already dreaming of margaritas on a sandy beach. We told ourselves it was a fair deal and decided not to dwell on it. Lesson learned.

Once the business was sold and our obligations settled, we did what any newly minted retirees would do—we bought a beachfront condo to renovate and declared ourselves officially retired. At 45, I thought I'd nailed the American Dream: retire early, enjoy life, and leave the rat race behind. For a while, we were busy updating the condo. Once we were satisfied with the renovation, we enjoyed endless beach days, lazy afternoons, and our suspiciously comfortable couch. Life was delightful! Unfortunately soon, the novelty wore off. Instead of feeling like a perpetual vacation, my days started to feel like a never-ending weekend with no Monday in sight. I became more restless, craving challenges and a sense of purpose. No one told me that eternal relaxation could start to feel like solitary confinement with better views.

At first, I relished the break. I soaked up the sun, went on long walks on the beach, devoured books, and had the time to really focus on my health. Yet the very absence of the 24/7 grind that had once seemed oppressive, now felt like an empty void. I missed the adrenaline rush, the daily challenges, and the sense of accomplishment that came from overcoming obstacles and finding new opportunities.

Determined to find my next big thing, I embarked on a journey of self-reflection. It was time to explore new avenues. I began looking inward and took a nostalgic stroll down memory lane, revisiting my past experiences and the skills I'd accumulated over the years. Surely, I could put them to good use. What have I done in my life? What skills do I possess? What experiences could I share?

Volunteering and mentoring seemed like a good place to start. I joined a non-profit organization dedicated to helping business owners and aspiring entrepreneurs navigate their paths to success.

Initially, it was a pragmatic decision. After all, how hard could it be to share a bit of wisdom and experience? I had no idea that this decision would come to hold profound personal and emotional significance, subtly transforming my outlook on life in ways that were as unexpected as they were gratifying.

When I began mentoring, I was met with a sea of eager faces, each one brimming with a mix of hope and apprehension. These were people at various stages of their entrepreneurial journeys, from the wide-eyed dreamers with ideas scribbled on napkins to the seasoned business owners facing new challenges. Their enthusiasm was infectious and stirred something deep within me—a long-dormant passion for teaching and guiding.

Soon, while working with my mentees, something magical happened. The act of mentoring transcended the mere exchange of knowledge. It became a two-way street of learning and growth. For every piece of advice I offered, I received insights in return—about resilience, innovation, and the sheer tenacity of the human spirit.

Mentoring was invigorating. I found myself in a familiar role, guiding eager entrepreneurs through the labyrinth of business management and ownership. I relished their "aha" moments and felt a sense of purpose returning to my life. I enjoyed sharing my knowledge and watching others grow their businesses. However, as rewarding as this was, through time, I noticed that I was repeatedly explaining and teaching the same business concepts. One mentee candidly said, "She wished everything was written down for her somewhere so she could read and re-read." Bingo! A light bulb went off, and I channeled my inner author; why not write a book? So I did. I poured my heart and soul into creating a comprehensive business plan book and workbook, a one-stop shop for aspiring entrepreneurs. Now, I had a comprehensive resource to share with my mentees for them to refer to on their own.

My book and workbook became my go-to tools during mentoring sessions. However, my enthusiasm for my materials eventually led to a little friction with the non-profit. They had their own materials and using my own resources created a conflict of interest. After some soul-searching, I decided to resign and continue mentoring independently. Free from any organizational constraints, I could use my materials as I saw fit and mentor on my own terms.

Despite the satisfaction mentoring brought, something still felt off. I was beginning to feel unfulfilled. My creative side was tugging at me, reminding me that writing a book was just the tip of the iceberg. There had to be more ways to unleash my creativity. I missed the thrill of creating something tangible, something I could see and touch.

As I pondered my next moves, reflecting on my career, I remembered my college days working in restaurants. Those were the days when I was young, broke, and full of dreams. After graduation, I was swamped with student loans and other expenses, so I turned my culinary skills into a catering side hustle. Eventually, I opened my own restaurant. Talk about biting off more than you can chew! But I was young and ambitious, and the restaurant business was a crash course in hard work and resilience, which gave me the confidence to start the next company in my 30's.

During my 20's, I got married, had a child, and eventually got divorced. As a single mom needing an affordable home, I met a real estate agent who became my mentor. He taught me the art of buying fixer-uppers, renovating them, and selling them for a profit. With my electrical engineering degree, I could read plans, understand building codes, and collaborate with contractors like a pro. Renovating homes turned out to be something I enjoyed. I got to be creative with interior design, constrained only by my budget, building codes, and the potential selling price. Flipping homes helped me pay off my student debt and fueled my creative fire.

Armed with this revelation and a drive to dive back into home renovation, I decided to go to design school to become a certified interior designer. This time, I wanted to do it right. It wasn't just about gaining credibility, but about refining my skills and expanding my creative toolkit. The coursework was demanding, but it reignited a passion within me. I was back in my element, balancing technical precision with creative freedom. The thrill of designing and renovating was addictive. I wasn't flipping houses; I was crafting dream homes. Each property presented unique opportunities and challenges, pushing me to think creatively and strategically. This was my sweet spot—combining creativity with the excitement of new challenges. Each project was a blank canvas, bringing fresh opportunities. I relished the challenges of dealing with the unknowns, negotiating with contractors, choosing fixtures and flooring, and finding the perfect shade of paint.

Stepping into an outdated home or condo for the first time is like opening the cover of an old, dusty book. You know there's a story hidden within, and with each turn of the page, each renovation decision, you're bringing that story back to life. The air is thick with potential, every cracked tile and faded wallpaper whispering secrets of a bygone era. My job, my passion, is to listen to those whispers and translate them into a modern symphony of design and functionality.

Imagine, if you will, the first impression of such a place. The door creaks open, revealing a dimly lit hallway lined with worn, once-plush carpet. The smell of aged wood and forgotten memories lingers in the air. It's here that I pause, not out of hesitation, but in anticipation of the transformation about to unfold.

Starting with the kitchen, often the heart of any home, this area is a relic from a past decade or more. With a once-vibrant vibe, it now resembles a patchwork of faded dreams. Here, the real magic begins. Tearing out these relics feels like shedding old skin. Out go the dated cabinets, making way for sleek, modern ones with clean lines and efficient storage solutions. Granite or quartz countertops replace the worn surfaces, their smooth, polished edges gleaming under new, strategically placed lighting.

Moving on to the other rooms, I'm beckoned to rejuvenate each one and seamlessly blend it with the modern updates. Fresh paint in soothing hues, new windows to let in natural light, and perhaps a cozy reading nook all transform these rooms into personal oases.

The exterior of the home is just as important as the interior. Curb appeal sets the tone for what lies within. A fresh coat of paint, updated landscaping, and new fixtures like a modern mailbox or house numbers can make a world of difference. Restoring the front porch, adding some comfortable seating, and maybe a swing turns it into a welcoming space that beckons visitors to sit and stay awhile.

Landscaping is the final brushstroke on the canvas. Overgrown bushes and neglected lawns give way to manicured gardens and lush greenery. Carefully laid paths lead to a serene backyard oasis complete with a patio or deck for entertaining, perfect for those warm summer evenings.

Each renovation is a dance between the old and the new, a delicate balance of preserving history and embracing modernity. It's about understanding the soul of the home and enhancing it with contemporary comforts and aesthetics. The process is as much about creativity as it is about construction - transforming spaces not just physically, but emotionally too. The final reveal is always worth the effort, a tangible manifestation of vision and hard work, ready to host new stories and memories.

After a few years, I began collaborating with custom home builders, renovating and designing new homes from the ground up. This added a new and welcomed challenge. I was able to fully utilize my creativity and solve problems in innovative ways. Renovating homes has always been a joy. This blend of technical skill and creative flair turned each project into a labor of love. The thrill of transforming outdated property into a dream home was unmatched for me.

Mentoring still plays a significant role in my life. I've found a way to balance it with my real estate ventures, offering guidance to aspiring entrepreneurs while indulging my creative side in home design. It's the perfect blend of giving back and staying engaged in something I enjoy. Through it all, I learned some valuable lessons that can help anyone on a similar path.

I've discovered that retirement isn't about slowing down. It's about finding new ways to channel your energy and passions. It's about stepping forward into new adventures, armed with the wisdom and experience of past endeavors. It's about finding joy in the journey, wherever it may lead.

Looking back, it's clear that my journey was anything but linear. I moved from business ownership to early retirement, volunteering and mentoring, and finally, returning to my true passion, home renovation and interior design. It's been a series of unexpected turns, learning experiences, and personal growth. Ultimately, selling my business wasn't the finish line I thought it would be. It was merely the starting point for a new chapter filled with creativity, challenges, and endless possibilities. And I wouldn't have it any other way.

As of now, I feel a sense of peace and contentment. My journey is far from over, but I'm excited for whatever comes next. Whether it's designing my next dream home, mentoring the next generation of entrepreneurs, or simply enjoying the beauty of each day, I know that I'm exactly where I'm meant to be.

CHAPTER 2

Trading Spreadsheets for Sunsets

"Time has this peculiar way of stretching and compressing,
especially when dreams take hold."

It feels like both a lifetime and the blink of an eye. Time has this peculiar way of stretching and compressing, especially when dreams take hold. I found myself often lost in visions of how I would run my own bed and breakfast. I can almost smell the fresh coffee brewing in the morning, see the sun casting golden rays over cozy, rustic rooms, and hear the soft murmur of satisfied guests enjoying a homemade breakfast spread.

The idea of owning a B&B became a cherished fantasy, inspired by tales from the 80s when bed and breakfasts surged in popularity. Back then, articles and books abounded with stories of couples who abandoned the hustle and bustle of city life. They fled to charming, picturesque locations like Vermont or Cape Cod, where they transformed quaint, historic homes into welcoming havens for travelers. Each narrative was filled with romance and adventure, detailing how these couples carved out a new, fulfilling livelihood in serene surroundings.

I imagined myself in those stories, walking through the rooms of my own charming inn, each space meticulously decorated with a blend of antique elegance and modern comfort. The garden would be a riot of color in the spring, with fragrant flowers lining the paths where guests could stroll leisurely. Evenings would be filled with the warmth of a crackling fireplace, as I shared local lore and personal anecdotes with visitors who soon felt like old friends.

These visions played out vividly in my mind, fueled by the dream of creating a space that isn't just a place to stay, but a memorable experience, a retreat from the everyday world where people could find peace and rejuvenation. This dream, sparked by those stories of 80s entrepreneurs, became a beacon that guided my ambitions and turned what once seemed like a far-off fantasy into a tangible, attainable goal.

But reality was upon me, stark and undeniable. My life bore no resemblance to that whimsical dream career of running a quaint bed and breakfast. Instead, I found myself entrenched in the bustling world of finance, working as a financial analyst in the heart of Boston for a massive mutual fund company.

My days were dominated by the hum and clatter of large, clunky computer screens that seemed almost monstrous in their size and noise, relics of an era when technology was more brute force than finesse. The HP 12C financial calculator was my constant companion, its worn buttons a testament to countless calculations. Hours were spent hunched over Lotus spreadsheets, their grids and formulas blending into a sea of numbers that demanded precision and focus.

As the sun set, my nights took on a different rhythm. The city lights of Boston blurred into a neon mosaic as I navigated the urban landscape. Pubs with creaking wooden floors and the comforting aroma of draft beer became my second home. There, the bartenders knew your name and your drink of choice - and the camaraderie of regular patrons provided a sense of community amidst the city's sprawling anonymity.

Despite the lively nightlife and the constant flow of conversations, there was a persistent sense of searching. Every evening was a new chapter in the ongoing quest to find my mate, that elusive partner who would understand my dreams and share in the adventures yet to come. The pubs were alive with laughter and stories, yet I often found myself caught in moments of introspection, wondering how far I had drifted from the life I truly wanted.

Amidst the financial reports and the social whirl, I clung to the daydreams of my B&B. The contrast between my daily reality and my nighttime reveries was stark. The Financial District's glass towers and the cozy, welcoming inn I had envisioned, were worlds apart. Yet, every spreadsheet completed and every pint shared brought me one step closer to the realization that my life, much like those stories from the 80s, could take an unexpected turn that would lead me to the peaceful haven I longed to create.

I did find my mate in one of those cozy, dimly lit Boston pubs. He stood out amidst the comforting chatter and the amber glow of aged wood and brass —a fellow traveler in the world of finance. He worked for a large Boston bank, extending loans to middle-market clients with the same meticulous care I applied to analyzing mutual funds. Our shared understanding of the financial world created an instant bond, and soon, we were inseparable.

We embraced city life with fervor, soaking up everything Boston had to offer. Our evenings were filled with the electric excitement of Bruins games, where the roar of the crowd and the clash of hockey sticks became a soundtrack to our budding romance. Summers brought us to the Boston Hatch Shell, where we sprawled on blankets and listened to symphonies under the open sky while the city skyline twinkled all around us.

Food became another of our shared passions and we often found ourselves wandering the cobblestone streets of the North End. There, we indulged in Italian feasts, savored rich, homemade pastas and enjoyed delicate cannolis- the flavors transporting us to another world. Each meal was a celebration of our life together and a testament to the joy we found in each other's company.

On weekends, we traded the urban hustle for the serene beauty of the northeast coastline. We walked along windswept beaches, the salty air tangling our hair and the sound of waves a soothing backdrop to our conversations. Boating became a favorite pastime of ours. The gentle rocking of the boat and the endless horizon fostered a sense of freedom and possibility. We lived for these moments as we embraced the simple pleasures of exploring new coves and watching the sunset paint the sky in hues of gold and pink.

Our life was a tapestry of these vibrant experiences, each thread adding depth and color to our shared story. The city of Boston, with its rich history and diverse offerings, became the backdrop to our love, shaping our days and nights in ways we had never imagined. However, throughout all those experiences, the dream of a bed and breakfast lingered, a quiet echo in the midst of our bustling lives. A constant reminder of the future we hoped to build together.

Those thoughts of owning a bed and breakfast never truly faded, always lurking in the corners of my mind. I often shared my dream with my husband, painting vivid pictures of our future inn nestled in a quaint, picturesque town. However, his reaction was always the same—a dismissive scoff followed by a gentle reminder of our current prosperity. He would say, "We have great jobs and everything we could want. Why trade it for a life of uncertainty?"

His reluctance was palpable. He wasn't the type of man who relished the thought of fixing clogged toilets or serving breakfast to strangers. The idea of waking up early to prepare a hearty meal for guests or spending weekends maintaining an old house held no appeal for him. He preferred the comfort and predictability of our urban lifestyle, where our roles as guests, not hosts, suited him perfectly.

While I dreamed of welcoming travelers with fresh-baked pastries and stories of local lore, he envisioned vacations where we were the ones pampered and catered to. The charm of a B&B, with its rustic charm and personal touches, clashed with his desire for luxury hotels and seamless service. My fantasies of sunny mornings spent chatting with guests over coffee and evenings by the fire with a glass of wine were met with his visions of a sophisticated city life.

Yet, I couldn't let go of the dream. It was like an itch that couldn't be scratched, a yearning that wouldn't be quelled. Every time we visited a charming coastal town or stayed at a cozy inn, I felt a pang of longing. I saw myself in the role of the innkeeper, creating a warm and welcoming atmosphere, sharing local secrets, and making each guest's stay truly special. My heart ached to transform a charming old house into a beloved retreat, where laughter echoed in the hallways and each room told a story.

Despite my husband's practical objections, the dream persisted, growing stronger with each passing year. The contrast between our visions of the future created an undercurrent of tension, a silent struggle between the stability of our present and the allure of a different life. My desire to build something uniquely ours—a haven of hospitality and charm—remained a constant, even as I navigated the bustling world of finance and city living.

In those quiet moments, as I watched the city lights twinkle from our brownstone window or strolled hand in hand through Boston's historic streets, the dream of a bed and breakfast whispered softly in my ear, reminding me of the life I yearned to create.

We never had kids. I suppose we were too wrapped up in the whirlwind of enjoying life, so immersed in each other and our careers that the thought of starting a family never quite took root. Our days were filled with the excitement of new experiences and the satisfaction of professional achievements, leaving little room for anything else. Twenty years flew by in the blink of an eye, and by then, we had become a mature couple—mature in our tastes, mature in our careers, and mature in our understanding of life.

Our home in the city evolved with us and eventually became a sanctuary of sophistication and comfort. We decorated it with pieces collected from our travels, each item a story and a memory: a handcrafted vase from a small village in Italy, an antique mirror from a Parisian flea market, and a vibrant painting from a local Boston artist. Our walls were adorned with framed photographs of our adventures, capturing moments of laughter, discovery, and love.

In our careers, we had climbed the ladders of success. I had moved up in the ranks at the mutual fund company, my office now boasting a stunning view of the Boston skyline. My days were filled with high-stakes meetings and complex financial strategies. My expertise and experience made me a respected figure in the industry while my husband achieved great success managing significant loan portfolios and becoming a trusted advisor to his clients.

Our professional lives were demanding, but they were also immensely rewarding. We found a rhythm that worked for us, balancing the pressures of work with the pleasures of our personal life. Evenings were often spent discussing the intricacies of our respective fields, sharing insights and advice over a carefully prepared dinner and a glass of wine.

Yet, amidst all this maturity and success lingered a dream of a bed and breakfast that never completely faded. It hovered in the background, a gentle reminder of a different path we could have taken. Sometimes, in the quiet of the night, I would imagine us in a quaint New England town. I could see us running our charming inn, welcoming guests from near and far, and creating a space filled with warmth and hospitality.

We were happy, deeply content with the life we had built together, but the dream of the B&B never left me. A constant "what if" that added a layer of complexity to our story. It was a testament to the dreams we held onto, even as life led us down different paths, shaping us into who we are and who we might still become.

One day, out of the blue, I was offered a buyout package. My firm was being acquired, a move that had been talked about in the hallways for months. While I knew the acquisition was imminent, I had always assumed I would be part of the new organization, continuing to climb the corporate ladder. Little did I know, that was not the plan. The news came as a shock, a jarring disruption to the steady cadence of my professional life.

As I sat in my office, staring at the offer letter, a swirl of emotions engulfed me. Surprise and uncertainty mingled with an unexpected sense of relief. Deep in my mind, I had known this change was for the best. I had become restless. My once steady dedication to my career waning in the face of an ever-growing whisper—a whisper that spoke of sunlit mornings in a quaint bed and breakfast, of and a vision of welcoming guests to a haven of comfort and charm.

That whisper had grown stronger over the years, becoming a persistent call that I could no longer ignore. Now, with this buyout package, I was being handed the opportunity to chase that dream. The financial security the package offered was substantial, enough to purchase an inn and have a cushion to support us through the transition. For the first time, I had both the money and the time to turn my long-held fantasy into reality.

However, one significant obstacle remained: convincing my husband. He had always been skeptical of my B&B dream, content with our urban lifestyle and the predictability of our careers. The thought of leaving behind the comfort and stability we had built together to venture into the unknown would be a hard sell.

That evening, as we sat in our beautifully appointed living room, the city lights casting a soft glow through the windows, I broached the subject. I spoke with passion, my voice trembling slightly with the weight of the moment. I told him about the buyout, how it was both an ending and a beginning. I painted a vivid picture of the life we could have, describing the charming inn we could create, the joy of welcoming guests, and the fulfillment of building something together.

He listened, his expression thoughtful. The skepticism was still there, but I could see a flicker of something else—curiosity, perhaps, or the stirrings of possibility. I spoke of the restlessness that had been growing within me, how my dream of the B&B had become a roar that I could no longer ignore. I explained that this was not just a dream, but a calling, one that I had to follow.

As the evening wore on, I could see him slowly warming to the idea. The feasibility of the buyout package, coupled with my steadfast conviction, started to win him over. We talked long into the night, exploring the possibilities, weighing the risks and rewards.

By the time we went to bed, there was a sense of tentative agreement. It wouldn't be easy, and there were many details to work out, but for the first time, the dream of our bed and breakfast felt within reach. The journey ahead was uncertain, but the excitement and promise of a new adventure filled me with hope. We were on the brink of a new chapter, ready to turn the page and embrace the unknown.

Together, we embarked on a quest that spanned several months, meticulously searching for the perfect house to transform into our bed and breakfast. The process was a journey in itself, filled with excitement, anticipation, and countless weekends spent exploring picturesque towns and scenic coastal areas. My husband, initially hesitant, soon found himself caught up in the thrill of the hunt. He reveled in scouting locations, assessing the architectural charm of potential houses, and scrutinizing prices to ensure we found the best deal.

Each visit brought us closer together, deepening our shared vision. We toured stately Victorian homes with their intricate woodwork and grand parlors, quaint cottages nestled by the sea, and sprawling farmhouses surrounded by rolling fields. We imagined our future in each one. We could picture guests arriving as rooms filled with laughter and warmth and the sweet scent of breakfast filled the air.

After months of searching, our perseverance paid off. We found our dream building in Chatham, Cape Cod—a quintessential Cape Cod home that seemed to leap straight out of a postcard. The house was perfect! It featured a charming, weathered exterior painted a soft yet inviting blue with white trim, a welcoming front porch adorned with wicker furniture, and a vibrant garden blooming with hydrangeas and roses. It stood proudly just off Main Street, close enough to the bustling heart of town, but secluded enough to offer peace and tranquility to our future guests.

The house boasted six spacious bedrooms, each with its own unique character. Some had quaint dormer windows offering views of the nearby sea, while others featured cozy reading nooks or antique fireplaces. The large yard was an oasis of greenery, with space for a vegetable garden, a patio for outdoor breakfasts, and a winding path leading to a secluded sitting area that was perfect for afternoon tea.

As we walked through the house, our excitement grew. We imagined each room lovingly decorated, blending antique charm with modern comfort. The living room, with its large bay window and inviting hearth, would become a communal space for guests to relax in and share stories. The dining room, where we envisioned serving hearty, homemade breakfasts, had a beautiful oak table that could easily accommodate a lively morning crowd.

My husband did not leave his job, maintaining his position at the bank while traveling to Chatham on weekends to assist with the renovations. This arrangement was part of our agreement. A compromise that respected the fact that while the bed and breakfast was my dream, it was not his. He enjoyed his work, thriving in the structured environment of finance and relishing the intellectual challenges it presented. The idea of running a B&B, with its unpredictable demands and the constant interaction with guests, didn't hold the same allure for him.

During the week, I delved into the transformation of our new home, managing contractors, selecting paint colors, and furnishing the rooms with a blend of antique finds and modern comforts. Each day brought a new set of tasks and triumphs. I spent hours scouring local shops for the perfect pieces to bring each room to life—a hand-carved headboard for the master suite, a set of vintage tea cups for the breakfast nook, and cheerful, floral fabrics for the curtains. The house slowly transformed into a welcoming haven with each room echoing the promise of future guests and shared memories.

My husband would arrive on weekends, bringing a mix of unwavering support and just enough pragmatism to keep me from doing anything too crazy. Despite his initial reservations, he took on the role of handyman with a surprising dedication, fixing leaks, sanding floors, and painting walls with meticulous care. We developed a rhythm to our weekends, working side by side during the day and relaxing in the evenings, often sitting on our front porch with a glass of wine, watching the sun dip below the horizon.

He might not have shared my enthusiasm for the B&B dream, but he supported it in his own way. We spent our evenings discussing our progress and planning the next steps, his analytical mind offering valuable insights and solutions to the challenges we faced. His commitment to our project, despite his own ambitions and reservations, deepened my appreciation for him. It underscored the strength of our partnership, our ability to support each other's dreams even when they diverged from our own.

As the inn began to take shape, we both found a sense of fulfillment in the work. For me, it was the realization of a long-held dream, a tangible manifestation of my passion for hospitality and comfort. For him, it was a testament to our shared journey and the life we were building together. The weekends became a cherished time, blending hard work with the simple joys of creating something meaningful and lasting.

By the time we completed the renovations, our bed and breakfast stood as a symbol of our combined efforts and dedication. The house was a blend of both our touches—his practical, sturdy improvements and my creative, welcoming decor. Each room was ready to welcome guests, from the cozy library filled with books and board games to the sunlit dining room where we would serve homemade breakfasts.

Despite the demanding weekdays apart, the weekends had cemented our bond even further, uniting us in a common goal. Our inn was more than just a business; it was a labor of love, a testament to our ability to navigate life's changes together. As we prepared to open our doors to the first guests, I felt a deep sense of gratitude for my husband's unwavering support and the adventure that lay ahead.

We finally opened the doors to our bed and breakfast, and I could hardly believe that the dream I had envisioned for decades had become a reality. The morning sun bathed our charming Cape Cod home in a golden glow as the garden was in full bloom, with vibrant flowers lining the pathways. The sign we had lovingly crafted swung gently in the breeze, proudly displaying the name of our inn.

Our first guests arrived with smiles and suitcases, and as I welcomed them, a surge of pride and excitement filled me. The house, now a warm and inviting haven, buzzed with the anticipation of new beginnings while each guestroom felt like a piece of my heart that was ready to offer comfort and hospitality.

However, the first morning was far from perfect. As our guests settled in, we quickly discovered the quirks and challenges of running a bed and breakfast. The hot water ran cold almost immediately as everyone decided to take showers at the same time. I could hear the confusion and laughter echoing through the halls and my heart sank momentarily. Thankfully, the guests seemed to take it in stride and made jokes about the brisk Cape Cod mornings.

In the kitchen, my plan for a seamless breakfast hit a few snags. The French toast I had intended to be golden and delicious came out slightly burned around the edges. The smell of overcooked bread mingled with the aroma of fresh coffee and I felt a pang of disappointment. My new employee, who was supposed to help with the morning rush, arrived late, looking flustered and apologetic.

Despite these hiccups, I put on a brave face and served breakfast with a smile, pouring coffee and chatting with our guests. To my surprise, they were incredibly understanding and gracious. They praised the homemade jams and complimented the cozy ambiance of the dining room. Their laughter and conversation filled the space, creating a warm and lively atmosphere that reassured me.

In my mind, the morning was a huge success. The little quirks and flaws only made our inn feel more inviting and authentic. I realized that while things might not always go as planned, the essence of my dream was alive and well. The guests felt welcome, the house was filled with life, and I was living the reality I had longed for.

Throughout the day, the inn continued to bustle with activity. Guests lounged in the garden, sipped tea on the porch, and explored the quaint streets of Chatham. In the evening, we gathered by the fireplace, shared stories and enjoyed the sense of community that had blossomed. My husband, though still more comfortable in his role as a supportive partner, joined in the conversations and his presence added a steady, reassuring warmth.

As I lay in bed that night, exhaustion mingled with a profound sense of fulfillment and accomplishment. All those years spent poring over financial statements couldn't compare to the satisfaction I felt now. A middle-aged woman with a decades-old dream had achieved what she set out to do. The dream was no longer just a dream; it was my life, with all its beautiful imperfections and unexpected joys.

Section 2 Introduction - Inspired

Many of the stories speak on a persistent ache that descends as disenchantment, a subtle yet insidious force. It whispers to them in quiet moments, reminding them of the dreams they once held dear and the paths they once hoped to tread. It casts a shadow over their achievements, leaving them wondering if the sacrifices they've made were truly worth it.

For some women, disenchantment manifested as a nagging sense of dissatisfaction with their careers. They may have climbed the corporate ladder, earned accolades, and garnered respect from their peers, yet deep down, they felt unfulfilled. The relentless pursuit of success left them feeling hollow, as if something vital was missing from their lives. Careers that once fueled passion and purpose, now felt like a never-ending grind.

For others, disenchantment took root in their relationships at home. They may have invested years in a marriage or partnership, some raising children, only to find themselves drifting apart from their significant other and their children. What was once a source of love and support had become a source of tension and discord, leaving them questioning the foundation upon which their relationship was built.

Then, there are those who felt disenchantment in the roles they had played out in their lives. The weight of responsibility they used to have may no longer be there, leaving a void in their lives and leading them to feel unfulfilled with what their daily lives now looked like.

Whatever the source of disenchantment may have been, its effects were universal. Many women's visions were clouded, temporarily distorting their perception of reality and obscuring them from seeing a path to fulfillment. Some were left feeling adrift in a sea of uncertainty, unsure of where they were going or even the possibility of getting there.

This pervasive sense of aimlessness often led to a profound sense of isolation, as if they were the only ones struggling with these feelings. The clarity of their ambitions and passions was dimmed, and many felt trapped in their routines, wondering how they would take the first steps toward the possibilities that awaited them.

Disenchantment was a subtle guidepost in each woman's journey of self-discovery. It was not a destination, but a signpost. It was the signal to their subconscious that something needed to change - that things were out of alignment with their true self. This realization often came with a mix of fear and excitement. The prospect of confronting these feelings head-on seemed daunting, but also presented an opportunity for profound growth and transformation. As they began to wake up to the possibilities of change, they started to question the assumptions and beliefs that had held them back.

CHAPTER 3

Twists, Turns, and Toffee

"You'll never have as much time as you do right now"

Ah, the timeless wisdom of aunts, they always seem to have a knack for dropping wisdom grenades when you least expect them. I remember when I was just a lively twelve-year-old, my aunt hit me with a truth bomb that still echoes in my mind today. She said, "You'll never have as much time as you do right now." And there I was, folding laundry like my life depended on it, itching to hit the tennis courts. Little did I know, she wasn't just talking about laundry; she was dropping some serious life advice.

Back then, time was just this annoying thing that made me late for dinner or made weekends end too soon. I didn't get it. Oh but how the tables have turned! In my teenage years, I was in such a rush to hit adulthood, thinking 21 was the magic number where life would finally "get real". Spoiler alert: it didn't. Then came the college rush, the career rush, the mid-life crisis rush. You name it; I was in a hurry to get there.

Somewhere amidst the chaos of adulthood, I realized I was playing life's game on fast forward. Suddenly, I hit my thirties, and time started slipping through my fingers like sand at the beach. I went from swinging rackets on the pro tennis circuit to shaking hands in the corporate world, then jumping ship to start my own consulting firm. Life was a whirlwind of suits, scenery, and self-discovery.

Then, just as I thought I had it all figured out, bam! The big 4-0 hit, and suddenly I'm feeling completely out of place. All my friends were married and had kids while I had neither a spouse or a child. The dinner conversations about child car seats and nursery school admissions were like foreign language broadcasts for me. In the blink of an eye, the notion of being single transformed from a deliberate lifestyle choice into an unexpected social anomaly, casting a new light on my place in the world.

I decided to take action in my quest for modern romance. I, like any forward-thinking individual, turned to the vast realm of the internet for guidance. With Match.com as my virtual haven, I delved into a digital landscape of profiles, swiping, and clicking my way through a myriad of options until I stumbled upon "Mr. CPA". Amid the digital sea of profiles, there he stood, his photo radiating a confident allure, clad in his office suit. His smile seemed to beckon, silently urging me with an unspoken invitation: "Choose me."

Let me tell you, diving into the world of online dating was like navigating a jungle filled with emoji-speaking monkeys and selfie-taking lions. Every profile was a potential adventure waiting to happen. As for "Mr. CPA", well, he may have been buried under a pile of paperwork, but his smile in that office photo spoke volumes. We exchanged emails faster than a cheetah chasing its prey. Before I knew it, I was contemplating whether love was truly a numbers game.

As I conversed with him, I couldn't help but feel like I was in a high-speed chat race, and he was winning by a landslide. Every word he uttered was like a precision strike, cutting through the fluff and getting straight to the point. I half-expected him to punctuate his sentences with a "TL;DR" (too long, didn't read), just to drive the efficiency point home. But in a world where time is money and brevity is the name of the game, his concise communication style was oddly refreshing.

So there we were, two adults navigating the treacherous waters of modern dating, armed with nothing but wit, charm, and a killer emoji game. That momentous night beneath the glittering cityscape soon arrived, where a simple invitation for drinks blossomed into an enchanting marathon of romantic dining.

As the evening unfolded, we found ourselves engrossed in conversation, effortlessly moving from deep, thought-provoking topics to light-hearted banter. Time slipped away, unnoticed, as we savored each moment. Our glasses clinking with each new topic we explored.

The cocktails we chose added an extra layer of enjoyment to our discussions. With names as intriguing as the flavors they held, they sparked curiosity and conversation. With each sip, we found ourselves delving deeper into the topics at hand, our laughter and shared stories filling the air around us.

In that moment, it felt as if time stood still, allowing us to fully immerse ourselves in each other's company and the delightful ambiance of the evening. Just when I thought the night couldn't get any more whimsical, he dropped the bombshell: a luxurious cruise invitation, complete with all the bells and whistles of a Hollywood romance.

Between the thrill of that unexpected invitation and the moment we stood at the cruise ship dock, the days blurred into a whirlwind of anticipation and blissful distraction. Every text message became a mini event, each plan meticulously designed to capture the essence of those heady early days. We found ourselves navigating the delicate dance of new love, a careful balance of excitement and vulnerability. Long conversations stretched into the early morning, where words flowed like wine, revealing dreams, fears, and everything in between. Stolen glances across candlelit dinners held the promise of something deeper, while spontaneous weekends away added a dash of unpredictability that kept us both on our toes. It wasn't always seamless, of course. There were moments when reality pierced through the fantasy, where misunderstandings or second-guessing brought us back down to earth. Love, even in its most dazzling form, had its cracks—times when we had to face the fact that this wasn't a fairy tale but something real, something that required patience, compromise, and trust.

Still, with each passing day, those bumps in the road felt less like obstacles and more like reminders that we were both in this together. As we got closer to the cruise, our excitement built with an almost electric intensity. What started as a casual fling had grown into something undeniably meaningful, and with every shared laugh or quiet moment, it became clear that we were ready to embrace whatever this romance would bring—no matter how unpredictable or wild the ride might be.

Three months later, there we stood, at the edge of the dock, our hearts pounding with a mix of excitement and nerves. We were about to embark on a voyage that would make Jack and Rose blush with envy.

As we stepped onto the deck of the magnificent cruise ship, hand in hand (because who has time for subtlety when you've got diamonds on your finger?), it hit me: this was it! The start of something beautiful, something wild, something that could only be described as a whirlwind romance on steroids. And so, with a twinkle in our eyes and a skip in our step, we set sail into the unknown, ready to conquer the high seas and each other's hearts. Love in the time of efficiency - who knew it could be so exhilarating?

Ah, the magical moment of matrimony - where two souls become one and daily routines suddenly become a team sport. I'll never forget the instant I said those two little words, "I do," and suddenly found myself hurtling headfirst into the abyss of shared responsibilities and synchronized schedules. It was like stepping through a portal into a parallel universe where "me time" became "we time" faster than you could say "honeymoon phase."

Before that pivotal moment, I was living my best solo life, blissfully unaware of anyone else's need for synchronized Google calendars or preemptive negotiations over who gets the last slice of pizza. It was all about me, myself, and I, basking in the warm glow of independence like a cat in a sunbeam. But alas, all good things must come to an end, and apparently, marriage was the end of my solo symphony and the beginning of a duet I never signed up for.

Then there were the wise words of my dear uncle, bless his brutally honest soul. "Good luck on taming her," he quipped to my husband, a sentiment that stung like a slap in the face at first, but in retrospect, was about as accurate as a GPS on a clear day. It was true I was about as wild and untamed as a herd of feral cats, and expecting me to suddenly morph into a domestic goddess overnight was like asking a sloth to run a marathon.

All of a sudden, I was navigating the choppy waters of matrimony like a reluctant sailor on the love boat. Adjustments? Ha! I had more adjustments than a chiropractor at a yoga convention. But, they say marriage is all about compromise, right? My free spirit got a crash course in the art of domestic diplomacy.

Marriage, I discovered, is like a perfectly choreographed dance routine; it's all about finding the right rhythm, mastering the steps, and occasionally stepping on each other's toes. It's a harmonious symphony of compromise, where you learn to blend your individual melodies into a beautiful duet. From navigating the quirks of morning routines to the art of sharing closet space, marriage requires a delicate balance of give and take. It's like being handed a puzzle with no picture on the box and figuring out how to make all the pieces fit together seamlessly. So, here's to the wonderful chaos of my marriage, where every adjustment is a step closer to mastering the ultimate pas de deux of love and partnership.

Yet, amidst the intricacies of marriage, it's crucial not to lose sight of individual passions and pursuits. Just as two trees intertwined their branches while still standing tall on their own roots, a thriving marriage embraces the growth and fulfillment of each partner. It's about nurturing the flame of personal ambition, while also tending to the shared fire of love and companionship. Striking this delicate balance requires open communication, mutual support, and a willingness to cheer each other on from the sidelines. After all, the most enriching marriages are those where partners not only walk hand in hand, but also encourage one another from the sidelines to chase their dreams, knowing that their shared journey is all the more vibrant for it.

As I crossed the threshold of 46, I found myself in a place of contentment, surrounded by the results of my career and the warmth of marriage and cherished relationships. Yet, amidst the comfort of routine and the familiarity of my accomplishments, there lingered a gentle whisper of longing for something more. It wasn't a dissatisfaction with my present, but rather a recognition of the untapped reservoirs of the potential within me. I knew that life was too precious to settle for the status quo, and my spirit yearned for new challenges, fresh adventures, and uncharted territories. With a quiet determination, I embraced the realization that my journey was far from over. That there was still much to explore, discover, and create in the chapters yet unwritten. For me, my 40s was not a milestone marking the end of possibilities, but rather the beginning of new and exciting chapters filled with promise and purpose. My aunt's words, "You'll never have as much time as you do right now," echoed in my mind, transforming into my newfound mantra.

I spent much of my youth with my grandmother, who stood tall with her gray hair tightly wound in a bun atop her head. Her presence was commanding, even intimidating to some of my friends, but her fondness for sweets softened her demeanor, bringing endless joy. With a passion for baking and cooking, she filled her home with the aroma of delectable desserts. Among her many specialties, toffee reigned supreme.

I can still recall the anticipation that would bubble within me as she embarked on her toffee-making ritual. The clinking of pots and pans, the rhythmic stirring, and the rich scent of caramelizing sugar filled the kitchen with an air of magic. With practiced hands and a heart full of love, she crafted each batch with care, infusing it with a warmth that transcended the ingredients.

The moment the toffee emerged off the stove, golden and glistening, was always met with eager anticipation. Its buttery richness and sweet crunch were a testament to her culinary prowess and unwavering devotion to making each treat a masterpiece.

Beyond the delicious flavors, it was the shared moments spent devouring her creations that remain etched in my memory. Gathered around the kitchen table, we would indulge in laughter and conversation, savoring each bite of her homemade toffee and the love that went into every morsel.

My grandmother's candy toffee recipe: a sweet legacy that started as a childhood lesson and evolved into a holiday sensation among my friends. They couldn't get enough of it! Some even joked that I should start selling it. Well, with my knack for toffee making and a craving for something more in life, I figured, why not turn this sugary skill into a sweet business venture? It was time to spread the sweetness beyond just my inner circle!

Entering the commercial food business was like diving headfirst into a culinary maze blindfolded, armed only with a spatula and a dash of determination. The fact that I knew as much about the food industry as a cabbage knows about calculus was oddly exhilarating. It was like setting sail on a ship without a map – terrifying yet thrilling. Every mistake was a lesson, every setback a spicy ingredient in the recipe of my education. I may have stumbled along the way, but isn't that the rhythm of mastering the cha-cha? With more than one kitchen catastrophe happening simultaneously, I was truly honing my skills.

Embarking on the journey of confectionery entrepreneurship felt like stepping into a whirlwind of sweetness, where each day unfolded with a flurry of lessons akin to a sugar rush – intense, rapid, and abundantly rich. While the cozy confines of my home kitchen had long been a sanctuary for experimenting with small batches of toffee, the leap to producing quantities fit for sale on platforms like HSN presented a formidable challenge.

As I immersed myself deeper into this sugary world, the complexities became apparent with every step. The transition from artisanal crafting to mass production demanded a profound shift in approach. It wasn't just about scaling up recipes; it was about mastering the intricacies of efficiency, consistency, and quality control on a whole new level.

One of the earliest lessons I encountered was the delicate dance of temperature control, especially as the Florida summer sun beat down mercilessly. Keeping the chocolate coating from melting into a gooey mess became an art form in itself. I found myself experimenting with various cooling techniques, from chilling rooms to specialized packaging, all in a bid to preserve the integrity of each delectable morsel.

It wasn't just about the chocolate, there were logistical hurdles to overcome, too. Procuring large-scale equipment was a daunting task that required meticulous research and strategic planning. From industrial-sized mixers to colossal tempering machines, each piece of machinery became a vital cog in the intricate machinery of my confectionery enterprise.

With each passing day, the learning curve seemed to steepen, yet the thrill of conquering new challenges fueled my determination. As I navigated the labyrinth of confectionery entrepreneurship, I realized that success in this realm wasn't just about satisfying sweet cravings; it was about mastering the delicate balance of artistry, innovation, and assembling a team to make every delectable bite.

In the bustling kitchen of life, I embarked on a journey to shake things up by curating a team as diverse and vibrant as a bustling spice bazaar on a lively Saturday morning. My vision was to orchestrate a symphony of talent, where the unique blend of experiences and opportunities would harmonize like ingredients in a meticulously crafted dish.

With this in mind, I sought out individuals who brought a kaleidoscope of perspectives and skills to the table. Among them were seasoned older women, their passion for culinary artistry undimmed by the passage of time and ready to showcase their expertise and vitality to the world. Alongside them stood autistic adults, their hunger for success matched only by their enthusiasm to leave an indelible mark on the culinary landscape.

It was akin to crafting the perfect recipe, each member of the team contributing their own distinct flavor to the mix. A pinch of resilience from those who had weathered life's storms, a dollop of determination from those striving to carve out their place in the world, and a generous measure of heart from all who shared a common goal.

Together, we stirred up a tempest in the candy world, breaking barriers and challenging conventions with every batch we crafted. Through our collective efforts, we not only crafted confections that delighted the senses, but also forged a path of inclusivity and compassion in an industry often marred by exclusivity.

For half a decade, I pursued my confectionery dream with the fervor of a child in pursuit of an ice cream truck on a scorching summer afternoon – relentless, unyielding, and propelled by an insatiable craving for success. However, much like savoring the final spoonful of a cherished dessert, I eventually reached a point where I could no longer stomach sacrificing yet another holiday to the relentless demands of the business. The holidays, once a time of joy and celebration, morphed into my own personal endurance test, engulfing every precious moment in a whirlwind of candy-coated chaos faster than one could utter the words "trick-or-treat."

After painstakingly building a spectacular team, perfecting our delicious offerings, and establishing a robust nationwide distribution network, I found myself standing at a significant crossroads. The idea of merely walking away felt inconceivable, as did the notion of selling our creation to a corporate behemoth, where its unique identity might vanish like sugar cubes melting into a cup of tea, leaving behind a bland uniformity.

Like many of us, I yearned for a legacy, something tangible to point to and proudly proclaim as my own. Without children of my own, I felt a deep need to create something that would outlast me. Over the past five years, I poured my heart and soul into building my business, knowing that it represented more than just a profit venture—it was a part of my family.

For me, the notion of legacy went beyond mere financial success; it was about leaving a mark, a testament to my hard work and dedication. I firmly believe in shaping one's destiny and being the author of one's own story. So, instead of letting my business fade into obscurity or be absorbed by a larger entity, I was determined to ensure its continuity and preserve its essence.

In doing so, I aimed not only to secure its future, but also to imprint my values and vision onto its legacy. This business was more than just a chapter in my life; it represented the culmination of my dreams and aspirations. It was a living testament to my belief in the power of forging one's own path and the importance of leaving behind a meaningful legacy. Each decision I made was infused with the intent to create something enduring, something that would speak to my commitment to excellence, innovation, and integrity. Through this endeavor, I sought to build a foundation that would inspire and guide future generations, ensuring that the essence of my values and vision would resonate long after I am gone.

I found a kindred spirit in one of our most treasured customers, the non-profit organization *Rethreaded*. We supplied our toffee to them, which they then private-labeled for their corporate fundraisers. *Rethreaded's* mission is deeply rooted in compassion and empowerment, embodying the principle of never turning away any survivor of human trafficking who seeks to rebuild their life.

At the core of *Rethreaded* lies a powerful belief in the transformative impact of secure and empowering employment. They understand that meaningful work not only provides financial stability, but also serves as a cornerstone for rebuilding confidence and strength in survivors of human trafficking.

Their commitment to offering survivors opportunities for dignified employment speaks volumes about their dedication to fostering resilience and facilitating long-term healing. By providing survivors with the means to support themselves and regain control of their lives, *Rethreaded* is actively shaping a future where every individual can thrive with dignity and purpose.

When *Rethreaded* approached me with an offer to purchase our toffee business, it felt like a perfect alignment of values and goals. It was a win-win scenario for everyone involved. For me, it meant passing on my grandmother's cherished toffee recipe to an organization dedicated to empowering women to rebuild their lives after escaping human trafficking.

Handing over the reins of the business ensured that my legacy would continue, not just as a successful enterprise, but as a force for positive change in the world. *Rethreaded*, in turn, gained a thriving operation that not only provided delicious treats, but also supported their mission of offering meaningful employment opportunities to survivors.

It was a moment of profound fulfillment, knowing that my entrepreneurial journey had culminated in a partnership that would leave a lasting impact on both the business world and the lives of those *Rethreaded* serves. Together, we were creating a legacy of empowerment, resilience, and hope.

If I hadn't heeded that gentle whisper urging me to continue creating or my aunt's words "You'll never have as much time as you do right now", I would have missed out on an abundance of experiences— the lessons learned, the invaluable insights gained, and the meaningful connections forged. Looking back, I'm filled with gratitude for embracing this journey later in life, when I could fully appreciate and savor every moment and opportunity it brought.

Each step of the way, I've discovered newfound depths of resilience, creativity, and determination within myself. The challenges I faced became opportunities for growth, and the setbacks only fueled my resolve to keep moving forward. Along the way, I've had the privilege of connecting with inspiring individuals, sharing stories, and learning from their journeys. My family and friends have been my bedrock, offering unwavering support and encouragement.

I also discovered that my husband is a keen marketer with an uncanny ability to articulate what our toffee eaters responded to in our branding. His insights turned out to be surprisingly spot-on. He once told me, "Honey, it's not just the toffee; it's the way it makes people feel." I initially thought he was just trying to butter me up (pun intended), but he was right. His knack for connecting with our customers' emotions has been invaluable. Plus, he's managed to turn taste-testing into grand adventures as we traveled across the state of Florida to all the Whole Foods and Lucky's Stores, sampling our toffees. Each store visit became an opportunity to meet new friends and toffee enthusiasts, sharing stories and laughs over bites of our sweet creations. We transformed mundane grocery store trips into exciting excursions, complete with impromptu tasting sessions and lively feedback exchanges. These journeys not only expanded our customer base, but also enriched our lives with unforgettable experiences and new friendships, proving that business can be both fun and deeply rewarding.

My aunt is the one who kept me calm during live nationally televised events. She would call ten minutes before I went on air to remind me to smile and have fun. She understood how stressed I was, and my husband was even more stressed since he was the one running the camera. It was during COVID, and all the live airings were done from our home kitchen. Now that was a true test of our marriage. Imagine trying to look composed on national TV while your spouse is whispering, "You're blocking the light!" and your aunt is cheerfully chanting, "Smile and have fun!" in your ear. Those moments not only tested our technical skills, but also reinforced the humor and love that keep us going.

Their belief in my potential has been a constant source of strength, bolstering my confidence during moments of doubt. Their wisdom and perspectives have enriched my understanding and opened my eyes to new possibilities. Their presence has been a guiding light, illuminating the path ahead and reminding me that I am never alone in this journey. The support of these cherished relationships has been the cornerstone of my perseverance, providing me with the emotional sustenance to navigate through every challenge and celebrate every triumph.

This late-life endeavor has been a testament to the power of embracing new beginnings and stepping outside of comfort zones. It's taught me the importance of staying open to possibility, even when it seems daunting or uncertain. Through it all, I've come to realize that the true beauty of creation lies not just in the end result, but in the journey itself—the moments of triumph, the lessons learned from failure, and the joy of simply being present for it all.

As I look back on this chapter of my life, I'm deeply grateful for the quiet nudges of inspiration and the unwavering support of my family that guided me forward, leading me to a journey of growth, fulfillment, and meaningful connections.

CHAPTER 4

A World Away, A World Within

"In the tangled web of childhood, I learned that even the darkest shadows can lead us to the brightest connections, where love and resilience illuminate our path forward."

I had always been a shadow in my own life, a silent observer on the fringes of my own story. Growing up with a bipolar mother cast a tumultuous shadow over my childhood, saturating it with uncertainty and chaos. As the eldest of three siblings, I bore the weight of responsibility from a tender age, stepping into the role of caregiver in a desperate attempt to shield my younger brother and sister from the tempestuous whirlwind of our mother's unpredictable moods.

Despite the turbulent backdrop of my upbringing, I remained resolute in my determination to carve out a stable life for myself. Upon graduating from college, my path intersected with David's in a serendipitous twist of fate. At first glance, David exuded an aura of charm and self-assurance, his easy smile and confident demeanor captivating my attention from the start. As our hearts intertwined, we embarked on a journey of love and companionship, swept up in the intoxicating whirlwind of youthful excitement and boundless dreams. Together, we envisioned a life brimming with love, laughter, and boundless promise.

However, as the years passed, cracks began to appear in the facade of our marriage. David's self-centered tendencies became more pronounced, his focus shifting increasingly towards his own needs and desires. I watched as he pursued his ambitions with single-minded determination, often at the expense of his relationships and the well-being of his family.

David's self-centered tendencies cast a shadow over my life, leaving me constantly walking on eggshells, never knowing when his next demand or outburst would come. His preoccupation with his own needs and desires created an atmosphere of tension and resentment within our home, suffocating my spirit and dampening my mood. I found myself constantly second-guessing my own thoughts and feelings, tiptoeing around David's fragile ego in an effort to avoid conflict. The weight of his expectations bore down on me like a heavy burden, draining me of the energy and enthusiasm I had once possessed. Despite my best efforts to maintain a facade of strength and composure, David's self-centered behavior eroded my sense of self-worth.. His behavior left me feeling invisible and insignificant in my own marriage.

Despite my growing dissatisfaction, I remained tethered to my marriage, anchored by a fragile thread of hope that whispered promises of change. I clung to the belief that with time, David would recognize the strain his self-centeredness placed on our relationship. That he would evolve into the partner I had once dreamed of. But as the days turned into weeks, and the weeks into years, that hope began to wane, leaving behind a hollow ache that gnawed at my heart.

In the midst of the tumultuous breakdown of my marriage, I discovered a sanctuary within the radiant presence of my two daughters, Emily and Sophie. Their laughter, like the tinkling of delicate chimes carried on a gentle breeze, filled the halls of our home, offering me a brief reprieve from the tempest swirling within me. With unwavering devotion, I poured my love and energy into nurturing them, finding solace in their innocent embrace and the boundless affection that flowed between them.

Within the refuge of those shared moments, I became a stalwart protector. Like a vigilant guardian, I shielded my daughters from the toxic undercurrents simmering beneath the surface of our household. I erected sturdy walls of protection around them, resolved to safeguard their childhood innocence for as long as humanly possible. Behind my warm smile, I concealed my own pain, sparing them from the burden of my troubles, steadfast in my belief that they deserved nothing less than the purest joy - untainted by the harsh realities of their surroundings.

Yet, even as I shielded my daughters from the harsh truths of their home life, I couldn't shake the nagging worry about the long-term impact of their upbringing. Would they, too, be condemned to a lifetime of navigating the treacherous waters of a fractured marriage? Or would they emerge unscathed, their spirits resilient against the shadows cast by their parents' strained relationship?

As I wrestled with these questions, I clung to the hope that my daughters would find their own paths to happiness and fulfillment, unencumbered by the mistakes of their parents. In quiet moments of reflection, I vowed to do everything in my power to ensure that their lives were filled with love, laughter, and boundless possibility, even if I couldn't find those same blessings for myself. Isn't that what every mother's greatest dream is?

However, as the years went by, I could no longer ignore the gnawing sense of emptiness that lingered within me. I watched as my own dreams and aspirations were overshadowed by the demands of my marriage and the expectations of society. The last thing I wanted was a divorce, but it seemed I was out of options. We had tried therapy, and while it seemed to help for a bit, I still felt suffocated by the confines of my marriage.

My days as an elementary school teacher provided me with a sanctuary away from the tumultuous currents of my personal life. In the classroom, surrounded by the eager faces of my students, I found a sense of purpose that transcended the chaos that awaited me at home. With each passing day, I poured my love and energy into nurturing the young minds entrusted to my care, guiding them with patience and compassion as they navigated the wondrous journey of learning and discovery.

The laughter that bubbled forth from my classroom became a balm for my weary soul, a reminder that even in the darkest of times, there was still light to be found. I reveled in the innocent curiosity of my students, their boundless enthusiasm a source of endless inspiration. Through their eyes, I glimpsed into a world brimming with possibility and wonder, a world untouched by the shadows that haunted my own existence.

Despite the joy I found in my work, I couldn't escape the persistent feeling of emptiness that lingered beneath the surface of my seemingly perfect life. Like a phantom limb, the void within me refused to be ignored. It gnawed at me from the inside with a relentless intensity that left me feeling hollow and adrift. No matter how hard I tried to bury myself in my work, the emptiness remained, a silent companion that followed me wherever I went.

As the years went by, I found myself questioning the choices I had made, wondering if I had taken a wrong turn somewhere along the way. I longed for a sense of fulfillment that seemed forever out of reach. I yearned for something more than the empty routine of my daily existence. In quiet moments of reflection, I couldn't help but wonder if I would ever find the courage to break free from the shackles of my own making. To reclaim the life I had lost somewhere along the way.

It wasn't until I reached my sixties, that I found the courage to confront the void within me. I realized that I had spent so much of my life tending to the needs of others that I had lost sight of my own identity. At that point I became determined to rediscover myself and I embarked on a journey of self-discovery that would change my life forever.

I soon realized that I had finally reached the end of my marriage. It was a decision that had been a long time coming and a culmination of years of emotional and psychological turmoil. I had been trapped in a relationship that had grown increasingly toxic through the years and what began with love and hope, had deteriorated into a constant state of tension and unhappiness.

My decision to end the marriage was not taken lightly. It involved endless nights of reflection, weighing the pros and cons, and coming to terms with the end of a significant chapter in my life. There was grief for what could have been, but there was also a growing sense of empowerment as I envisioned a future free from the toxicity that had held me captive.

Deep inside I knew I no longer needed or wanted to be part of a marriage that suffocated me. I yearned for peace, for a space where I could breathe freely and rediscover myself. The final decision to leave wasn't easy, but it was necessary. I had to prioritize my well-being and reclaim my life from the shadows of our broken relationship.

As I packed my belongings, each item was a reminder of the life we had built together and the dreams that had faded over time. There were moments of doubt, moments where the fear of the unknown almost paralyzed me, but the thought of staying in a loveless, toxic marriage was more terrifying. I deserved more—I deserved happiness, respect, and the chance to rebuild my life on my own terms.

Looking back, the signs had been there for a long time. Arguments we never seemed to be able to resolve, cold silences that stretched between us, and a pervasive feeling of walking on eggshells in my own home. The love that once bound us had withered away and was instead replaced by resentment and a deep sense of loss. Each day felt like a battle that drained away my spirit and left me feeling isolated and unseen.

Leaving the marriage meant starting over, but it also meant rediscovering myself. The decision was a daunting leap into the unknown, but it was also liberating. I was no longer defined by the oppressive dynamics of a broken relationship. Instead, I was free to explore my passions, dreams, and aspirations that had been stifled for so long. It was a journey of self-discovery, filled with moments of both vulnerability and strength.

I began to reconnect with hobbies that once brought me joy. Painting, which had been abandoned in the midst of marital strife, became a therapeutic outlet. Each stroke of the brush on the canvas felt like a step towards reclaiming my identity. I started writing again, pouring my thoughts and experiences into journals that captured my evolving sense of self.

Traveling became another avenue of self-exploration. I visited places I had always dreamed of, from serene beaches to bustling cities, soaking in the beauty and diversity of the world. Each destination offered new experiences and insights, helping me to rebuild my confidence and broaden my horizons. However, traveling alone was not without its challenges.

Navigating unfamiliar territories tested me in ways I hadn't anticipated. From the very first step into a bustling foreign city, I was thrown into a whirlwind of new experiences, each one more challenging than the last. The language barrier was one of the first hurdles—signs in foreign scripts that seemed like riddles, street names that twisted my tongue, and the constant struggle to make myself understood. Even something as simple as ordering a cup of coffee felt like an obstacle course, as I tried to decipher menus in a language I couldn't read and communicate my basic needs with hesitant gestures. The words I knew seemed inadequate in the face of such complexity, and I was left to rely on my ability to observe, to listen, and to piece together meaning from context.

Then came the public transportation systems—each city had its own maze of buses, trains, and subways, all running on schedules that felt like a puzzle waiting to be solved. I would stand at the edge of a crowded metro station, map in hand, trying to figure out which train to board and whether I needed to make a transfer in a city where I didn't speak the language. There were moments when I got on the wrong train, only to be whisked away to an unfamiliar part of town, wondering if I would ever find my way back. But rather than feeling defeated, I found myself growing more resourceful with each misstep. I began to trust my instincts, using landmarks, a rudimentary knowledge of the city's layout, and the kindness of strangers who would occasionally offer help, even when I could barely understand their words.

In those moments of feeling lost—whether physically or mentally—it was as though I was shedding layers of old fears and doubts. There was a certain freedom in embracing uncertainty. I learned to laugh at my mistakes and see them as stepping stones rather than setbacks. Each obstacle became an opportunity to stretch my limits and push past the discomfort of the unknown. I could feel my confidence growing with every challenge I faced, like a muscle that strengthened the more it was tested.

One particular experience stands out: I was in a small town in Italy, trying to find my way to a remote village for a hiking trip. The train I boarded was delayed, and I missed my connection to the bus that would take me up the mountain. There I was, standing in an empty station late in the evening, with no clear way forward. But rather than panicking, I remembered something my grandmother once told me: "When in doubt, ask someone." And so I did—asking a local shopkeeper who spoke no English for directions. He smiled, nodded, and with a series of hand gestures and broken words, managed to communicate that I could walk the rest of the way to the village. It was a 45-minute uphill trek, and I had no idea what I would find at the top, but I decided to take the leap.

As I walked through narrow, winding streets under the warm golden light of a setting sun, I marveled at how far I had come—from feeling lost and isolated to finding my way through a foreign land. By the time I reached the village, tired but elated, I had learned an invaluable lesson:

that discomfort is often the birthplace of growth, and that our ability to adapt and think on our feet is what makes us resilient in the face of life's challenges.

Each misstep, each moment of uncertainty, became a building block of self-reliance. I had learned that not knowing exactly where I was going didn't mean I couldn't get there—it just meant I had to trust in the process, trust in my ability to navigate through the unknown. And with that trust came a profound sense of accomplishment, one that stayed with me long after I had returned home. It was a reminder that stepping outside of our comfort zones, no matter how intimidating, is always worth the journey.

I learned how to find safe and comfortable places to stay, often by relying on the recommendations of fellow travelers or online reviews. Each new place required an adjustment period as I figured out the best local eateries, markets, and attractions which sometimes led to unexpected adventures like staying in a quirky hostel where I made lifelong friends or a serene bed-and-breakfast that offered the perfect escape.

Meeting new people along the way was both a joy and a challenge. It required making an effort at initiating conversations and being open to different perspectives. Each new encounter enriched my journey, whether it was a fellow traveler sharing their own stories of self-discovery or a local offering insights into their culture and way of life.

While I met many wonderful people in my travels, I also spent many evenings dining alone, surrounded by the hum of conversations in languages I couldn't understand. These solitary moments became opportunities for introspection and growth. I learned to enjoy my own company, to find peace in the quiet, and to appreciate the freedom to chart my own course without compromise.

Despite the hurdles, traveling alone gave me the confidence I needed. For so many years I had been stripped of it, feeling as though I had lost a part of myself that I might never reclaim. Each challenge—navigating new cities, overcoming language barriers, and managing solitary moments—became a stepping stone toward rediscovering my self-assurance. As I faced and conquered these obstacles, I began to realize that the confidence I thought was lost forever was slowly being rebuilt, bit by bit. Each successful adventure and new experience fortified my belief in my own capabilities, proving to myself that I was far more resilient and resourceful than I had ever imagined.

I also invested time in my personal growth. I attended workshops and seminars on topics ranging from self-care to entrepreneurship, eager to learn and evolve. These experiences empowered me and provided me with the knowledge and tools I needed to build a future on my own terms.

Another critical aspect of my journey was having the chance to form new relationships. I met people who appreciated me for who I truly was, free from the shadows of my past. These connections, whether fleeting or lasting, added richness to my life, and reinforced my belief in the goodness and potential within me.

Don't get me wrong, there were moments of vulnerability where the weight of starting over felt overwhelming, but these were counterbalanced by moments of incredible strength. Moments where I realized just how resilient I had become. Each day, I grew more confident and self-assured, piecing together a life that was not only functional, but deeply fulfilling and true to who I was.

Physically, I felt the effects of age, but I also knew that taking care of my body was more important than ever. I embraced a healthier lifestyle, incorporating regular exercise and nutritious eating habits into my daily routine. Yoga and meditation became essential practices that helped me maintain balance and inner peace. The physical and mental strength I gained from these practices was instrumental in my ability to face challenges head-on.

Emotionally, I learned to let go of the guilt and self-doubt that had plagued me for so long. Therapy and support groups were invaluable in this process, providing a safe space to express my feelings and receive guidance. I realized that it was never too late to heal, to grow, and to find happiness. My age did not define me; my actions and choices did.

In this new chapter of my life, being older was not a hindrance, but a powerful advantage. I approached each day with the wisdom of my past experiences and the courage to embrace the unknown. The years behind me were filled with lessons that strengthened my resolve and sharpened my vision for the future. I was not just surviving; I was really experiencing and living, proving that it is never too late to shift your narratives and write a different chapter than you imagined.

Section 3 Introduction - Encouraged

Each woman's initial stride toward reclaiming their sense of purpose and joy was to shift their perspective. Instead of viewing disenchantment as permanent, they chose to see it as a catalyst for change. They recognized that their current circumstances did not define them, and that they had the power to create the life they wanted to live. Not knowing where their journey might lead them, many found answers in unexpected places, hidden beneath layers of conditioning and societal expectations. Disenchantment was not the end of the road; it was the beginning of a new chapter. It was the wake-up call, the reminder that they were the authors of their own destiny. The path ahead may have seemed uncertain, but it was also filled with infinite possibilities and opportunities.

Their awakening and acceptance of exploration often involved a gradual process of introspection and self-discovery. They started to pay closer attention to the small sparks of joy and curiosity in their daily lives, now recognizing them as clues to what they truly valued and desired. They began to envision a life that aligned more closely with their passions and dreams, rather than one dictated by external expectations or obligations. This new awareness opened pathways for them to explore, breaking down the mental barriers that had previously kept them confined.

This shift in perspective pulled them to embrace a sense of curiosity and openness. By quieting the chatter of their minds and tuning into the present moment, they worked to cultivate a sense of inner peace and clarity. Rather than dwelling on what was wrong in their lives, they began to explore the realms of fulfilling possibilities. They embarked on a journey of self-discovery, asking:

What do I truly value in life?
What brings me joy and fulfillment?

What are my wildest dreams and aspirations?

What steps can I take to bring those dreams to fruition?

By reframing their thoughts this way, they opened themselves to new possibilities and opportunities. They began to see disenchantment not as a roadblock, but as a stepping stone on the path to a more fulfilling existence. Ultimately, disenchantment became a powerful catalyst for self-discovery and empowerment. It encouraged them to reassess their lives, make meaningful changes, and embrace the possibilities that laid ahead. By listening to and acting upon this inner signal, they embarked on a transformative journey that led to a more authentic, fulfilling existence.

Once they embraced their new perspective, they understood that knowing what they wanted was simply not enough. They had to take action to bring their dreams to fruition. They stepped out of their comfort zones, not searching for the right answers, but listening to the whispers of their hearts. Initially, some felt hesitant or fearful when faced with the prospect of stepping into the unknown, but they ultimately felt ready to stretch and challenge themselves to reach their full potential.

CHAPTER 5

The Hollow Steps to Wholeness

"In the delicate dance of reconnection, I discovered that vulnerability is not a weakness, but a profound strength that rethreads the heart."

Countless mornings blurred together, each beginning with tear-soaked pillows and a heart weighed down by sorrow. After 32 years of marriage, the pain of separation felt unbearable. For my entire adult life, I had been the other half of a couple, until now. I had heard the term "heartbreaking" before, but it was only now that I truly grasped its meaning. Hearts can indeed shatter into pieces. Perhaps it was the deep connection and interlacing of our lives that made me feel like my heart had been broken into fragments, but all I knew at that moment was that I was shattered.

In truth, it wasn't a sudden halt, but rather an eleven-month journey of unraveling. We found ourselves immersed in waiting rooms, buried beneath piles of medical forms, clinging to every "we can try" as if it were a lifeline. We prayed fervently for a magic pill to cure the cancer, each attempt laden with the weight of our desperate longing for a miracle. Yet, as the months stretched on, the attempts became scarce, dwindling to almost nothing in the final three months.

We held onto each other, finding solace in the belief that tomorrow would bring relief. Our family and friends rallied around us, offering nourishment, and fleeting moments of normalcy from the outside world. Despite our efforts to maintain a sense of normalcy, participating in birthday celebrations felt hollow when the shadow of uncertainty loomed over us, casting doubt on the possibility of another celebration.

We made a conscious effort to conceal our fear and pain, shielding it even from ourselves. For me, the beach became a sanctuary, a place where I could release my pent-up emotions, letting tears mingle with the salty waves. I walked for miles, attempting to compose myself, to bury those feelings deep within, hoping they wouldn't resurface for anyone to see.

As the end grew near, both family and friends offered comforting words such as: "He is fighting so hard." Deep down, I knew these words held truth but despite my best efforts to push it away, I could feel the inevitable approaching.

When the day finally arrived, it was as if my heart had not been preparing for it all along. That sadness came with an overwhelming sense of paralysis, moments where I felt incapable of moving, as if the weight of the world had pinned me down. There were times when even drawing a breath felt like an insurmountable task. My life ground to a halt so suddenly that I feared it might never restart again.

I found myself submerged in a sea of darkness, enveloped by feelings of depression and despair that seemed to emanate from within me. Despite the well-meaning attempts of family and friends to offer words of encouragement such as "tomorrow will be better" and "take it one step at a time," I found it challenging to focus on anything beyond the overwhelming emotions I was grappling with at the moment. The weight of my struggles felt insurmountable, casting a shadow over any glimmer of hope or positivity that others tried to impart. Each day seemed like an uphill battle, and the prospect of a brighter tomorrow felt distant and unattainable as I navigated through the depths of my emotions.

The innocuous inquiry, "Are you going to put the house up for sale?" elicited an involuntary cringe within me. While on the surface, the status of the house may have seemed like a straightforward matter to address, it paled in comparison to the weightier decision that loomed over me each day. What laid at the core of my being was not a matter of real estate transactions, but rather daunting questions like whether I could muster the strength to emerge from the confines of my bed and face the world by simply getting dressed.

I was trying to navigate my new reality. The external world appeared distant and inconsequential in comparison to the conversations raging within my mind and heart. The mere act of contemplating the sale of a house seemed trivial when juxtaposed against the monumental task of confronting my inner struggles and finding the courage to engage with the world. Each day presented an intimidating challenge. I had to grapple with the profound uncertainty of my own circumstances, all while concealing the depth of my inner turmoil from the casual observers around me.

The fog of confusion and disorientation that enveloped me seemed to reach its peak around the two-week mark. It was during this time that everyone around me began to resume their normal routines, while I found myself adrift in a sea of uncertainty. My own familiar routine had vanished, leaving me with a profound sense of emptiness and a daunting question mark hanging over my future. The reassurances that time would heal were offered to me, yet I couldn't shake the overwhelming doubt of whether I possessed the strength and resilience to rebuild my life from the ground up.

The shift from being part of a couple for 32 years to facing the reality of being single felt like an insurmountable mountain. The thought of navigating this uncharted territory and reshaping my identity from a duo to a solitary individual weighed on me like an overwhelming burden. How does one untangle the intricacies of shared lives, memories, and dreams built over decades? The prospect of forging a new path forward seemed both daunting and uncertain. I was left wrestling with self-doubt and a profound sense of inadequacy. The road ahead loomed large, with no clear map to guide me through the uncharted terrain of newfound solitude.

The collection of grief books on my nightstand seemed to multiply with each passing day, forming a towering testament to the profound pain and loss that had taken root in my life. Despite the efforts of well-meaning friends who encircled me with their support and encouragement, gently nudging me towards the path of healing, I found myself steadfastly anchored to the past and unwilling to relinquish the memories that had become my lifeline.

As the days stretched into weeks, the weight of those memories bore down on me like a heavy shroud, casting a shadow over my every waking moment. The memories wove themselves into the tapestry of my existence, coloring my thoughts, feelings, and dreams with shades of nostalgia and longing. The past, with all its joys and sorrows, unfolded before me like a vivid tableau. Each memory, a bittersweet reminder of a life that once was.

In the quiet hours of the night, when the world slumbered and my thoughts roamed free, the echoes of the past reverberated through my mind, mingling with the whispers of my dreams. The line between waking and sleeping blurred as the boundaries of time and memory dissolved. I would find myself adrift in a realm where the past and present converged in a dance of remembrance and reflection. Amidst the solace of solitude, I sought refuge in the familiar contours of my memories, clinging to them as if they were fragile lifelines keeping me afloat in a sea of uncertainty and grief.

The gradual realization of my profound sense of loneliness and solitude unfolded like a silent storm, devoid of a distinct moment or clear demarcation in time. Days blurred into nights, and weeks melted into months, as I navigated the murky waters of my own isolation. While I maintained a semblance of normalcy by engaging in social activities with friends, the truth was that I was merely going through the motions as a ghostly presence amidst the lively chatter and laughter that surrounded me. Physically present, but emotionally distant. I found myself adrift in a sea of my own making, grappling with the weight of my unspoken sorrows and unmet needs.

The realization unfolded within me gradually, like the hesitant tendrils of light piercing through the veil of darkness at dawn, gradually illuminating the cavernous depths of my solitude with a profound clarity. It marked not just a moment of reckoning, but a somber awakening to the profound disconnect that had stealthily draped itself around me, weighing heavily like a suffocating cloak upon my shoulders.

I started to fill my calendar with mahjong, bridge, and a luncheon every week. Despite the outward veneer of camaraderie and companionship that adorned my social interactions, I found myself drifting aimlessly in an expansive sea of emptiness. In the midst of the noise created by shallow exchanges and surface-level connections, a quiet longing began to stir within me—a desire for authentic understanding and meaningful human connection that went beyond the emptiness of daily interactions.

As I reflect upon the meaningless nature of my interactions and the echoing emptiness that pervaded my days, I knew deep within my soul that a change was necessary. The path to healing lay in rekindling the flames of connection, in reaching out beyond the confines of my own solitude to forge meaningful relationships and shared experiences. The road ahead was fraught with uncertainties and vulnerabilities, but I understood that it was a journey I needed to undertake in order to ease the ache of loneliness and rediscover the joy of genuine human connection. Embracing this newfound awareness as a catalyst for change, I resolved to step out of the shadows of my isolation and into the light of reconnection. I knew that the journey towards healing and wholeness would begin with a single step.

The process of emerging from my shell of isolation was not a sudden, drastic transformation. Instead, it unfolded gradually, like the delicate unfurling of a flower bud in the early light of dawn. Each step forward felt like the slow turning of a key in a rusty lock, coaxing hesitant progress as slivers of light filtered through the cracks of my solitude.

The decision to join a support group was a pivotal moment, one that required summoning courage I didn't know I possessed. Walking into that room for the first time felt like stepping into the unknown, as if I were stepping off the edge of a cliff and trusting that the air itself would hold me. My vulnerability felt raw and exposed, like a delicate wound freshly uncovered, throbbing with the awareness of being seen.

The room was simple, unassuming—plastic chairs arranged in a circle, a faint scent of coffee lingering in the air, and a table in the corner stacked with pamphlets and tissues. Yet, it buzzed with an unspoken energy, a blend of apprehension and hope that seemed to pulse beneath the surface. The faces I saw were etched with a familiar heaviness, a quiet determination to be there despite the weight of their own burdens.

When I sat down, my heart pounded like a drumbeat echoing in my ears. My hands gripped the edges of the chair, as though anchoring myself in the moment could keep the tide of uncertainty from sweeping me away. The introductions began, each voice hesitant at first, then growing steadier as stories spilled into the space between us.

What I found there was not judgment but acceptance, a quiet nod here, a warm smile there, gestures that spoke louder than words. The shared stories wove themselves into a tapestry of collective strength, each thread carrying its own distinct color of pain, hope, and resilience. Some voices trembled as they recounted their loss, while others carried the steadiness of someone who was starting to recover from their loss.

It was in those moments that I realized connection didn't require perfection or eloquence. It demanded only presence—the willingness to sit with one another's truths, to bear witness without trying to fix or diminish the weight of what was shared. The air seemed to grow lighter with every story, not because the sadness disappeared, but because they were no longer alone.

While our struggles were unique, our desire for connection was universal, a thread that bound us together even in our differences. The room became a sanctuary, a place where I could finally begin to release the walls I had built so carefully around myself. And as the meeting came to an end, I walked out feeling a little less alone, as if the first stitch in my own unraveling isolation had been sewn.

As the weeks turned to months, I became more attuned to the subtle changes taking place within and around me. Like a tender sapling stretching its leaves towards the sun, I tentatively reached out to embrace the possibilities that lay beyond my comfort zone. Every hesitant step forward I took as I navigated the uncharted territory of vulnerability made me aware of the fragility of my healing spirit - yet emboldened me with the glimmers of resilience that flickered within.

In this profound journey of self-discovery and connection, I found myself assuming the role of both student and teacher. I had to learn the intricate steps required to reach out and forge bonds with others. Every interaction, no matter how fleeting, assumed significance as a lesson in vulnerability, empathy, and the intricate tapestry of human connection.

As I navigated the labyrinth of reconnection, I discovered that this process was not merely a series of external actions, but a deeply personal and introspective odyssey. Each chapter is a reflection of my own inner growth, unfolding at a pace uniquely tailored to my needs and experiences. With each encounter, I unearthed layers of understanding, honing my ability to empathize and connect with those around me in a way that felt authentic and profound.

I realized that there is no one-size-fits-all approach to healing and rebuilding connections after a period of isolation. Each individual approaches this journey on their own terms, guided by their own inner compass and shaped by their personal experiences and circumstances. Just as I had embarked on my own path of self-discovery and growth, I understood that others would also navigate their own journeys of reconnection in ways that resonated with their hearts and souls.

I immersed myself in the beauty of imperfection, recognizing that growth often emerges from the fertile soil of vulnerability and authenticity. In this sacred space of shared humanity, I discovered the profound wisdom that accompanies the willingness to lean into discomfort and uncertainty, finding strength in the delicate balance between courage and vulnerability.

After what seemed like a lifetime to me, I found myself ready to reemerge into the world and embark on the journey of establishing a new routine. Though my heart had been mended, it still bore the scars of loss that served as a poignant reminder of the life I had once known. Yet, with each passing day, these scars, both physical and emotional, began to gradually fade away, much like the tears that once flowed freely.

I still see myself as part of a duo, but I've come to realize that I can thrive on my own. The memories, rich and vivid, have been transformed into memories of shared experiences and cherished moments. These recollections have softened the pain and also provided a comforting reminder of the strength and resilience I've gained along the way.

CHAPTER 6

Watercolors and Baby Steps

"In a single moment, my world unraveled, leaving me feeling invisible and adrift, as the dreams of a united family faded into the stark reality of loss and uncertainty."

In a single, heart-wrenching moment, my world unraveled. The vision I had clung to of a united, ever-happy family crumbled into the harsh reality of loss and uncertainty. Dreams don't end with a neat little bow — they unravel messily.

It happened one unassuming afternoon. He came over with the kids, wearing the kind of expression that makes your stomach drop before a single word is spoken. Then, with a tone as casual as if he were ordering coffee, he said, "The kids are going to live with me now, and you have to pay child support."

Wait—what? I blinked. *What just happened?* Then, as if it were nothing at all, he left—with *my* kids. My heart and my sanity walked out that door with them. I protested, of course. I begged, "Tell me what to do, and I'll do it!" But they had no answers. This truly shocked me to my core. I could not believe I had ended up here.

This wasn't just jarring—it was as if someone had taken my life, tossed it in a blender, and hit "purée." I felt ridiculous. How had I ended up here, blindsided and unmoored? Just a month ago, we'd finalized the divorce. I thought everything was settled, that we were the poster children for "amicable co-parenting." I actually believed we were special—capable of weathering anything together.

No, I was no longer part of the plan. I was left floundering, crying my way through days that blurred together like watercolor paintings left out in the rain.

For nearly two decades, I'd been a stay-at-home mom. It was my life, my identity, my joy. My ex's global travel schedule left little room for me to pursue anything outside of the home. And honestly, I didn't mind. I loved being there for the kids, for every milestone, every scraped knee, every sleepy bedtime story. I thought we were a team. Apparently, I missed the memo that we were only playing the first half.

So, there I was: an empty nester *years* before I ever expected to be, with no job, limited savings, and no clue what to do next. For at least a year, I was a ghost of myself—wandering, ruminating. stuck in a loop of self-doubt. I barely remember that time, except that it was boring, lonely, and tinged with panic.

I kept telling myself I'd "go back to school one day," or "reconnect with my old colleagues," but I hadn't done either. Now, it felt too late. The future loomed ahead like a giant question mark, and I was too paralyzed to even attempt to answer it.

But then, one day, I stumbled across a book: *What Color is Your Parachute?* It asked questions like, "What makes you lose track of time?" and "What doesn't feel like work?" These questions sparked something in me—a flicker of curiosity in a sea of hopelessness.

I started to reflect. I loved working in public health before the kids. I adored working with children. And I had a hobby of making mosaics that brought me joy. But how could I make a career out of any of that?

Mosaics were quickly ruled out (as much as I loved them, "starving artist" wasn't on my bucket list). Public health intrigued me, but the pay wasn't great, and I needed something sustainable. Then, a light bulb went off: *newborn care.* It was the perfect intersection of everything I loved– babies, nurturing, and even a touch of public health.

I spent months researching, planning, and dreaming. A friend had a baby around this time, and she became my first "client," helping me work out the kinks of my fledgling idea. I was giddy with excitement. Imagine getting *paid* to hold babies all night while their parents caught up on sleep!

But there was a catch. To get clients, I needed to network—reach out to friends, neighbors, and acquaintances. This terrified me. I worried they'd see me as desperate or, worse, pity me. I spent *weeks* agonizing over how to approach them.

Finally, I swallowed my pride and reached out. And guess what? They were thrilled for me. They didn't see me as "the help." They saw me as someone passionate and capable, and they were eager to support me. I wish I hadn't wasted so much time worrying about their reactions.

My work became deeply fulfilling. Most of my clients were first-time parents, overwhelmed and sleep-deprived. I'd swoop in, offer guidance, and help them navigate the rollercoaster that is the newborn phase. I'd stay overnight, rocking their little ones under the soft glow of the moon while they got some much-needed rest.

At first, I missed the creative outlet I thought I'd sacrificed. But soon, I found ways to bring creativity into my work—designing colorful schedules, crafting watercolor notes for parents, and even creating art that hung in their nurseries.

Now, I often find myself in the still of the night, holding a baby as the world sleeps, marveling at how far I've come. "I can't believe I get paid to do this," I think, smiling to myself.

Life threw me a curveball, but I didn't just catch it—I turned it into something beautiful. What felt like an ending was really a new beginning.

And you know what? That's good for my soul! Job well done, me.

CHAPTER 7

Divine Grace After the Storm

"Each day in that dark world stripped away pieces of my identity, leaving behind a hollow shell where my hopes and dreams once flourished."

My story is just like that of countless other women who have fallen victim to the sex trafficking industry. It is a tale marked by incredible loss—loss of direction, loss of self, and the devastating loss of everything that once defined my life. Each day in that dark world stripped away pieces of my identity, leaving behind a hollow shell where my hopes and dreams once flourished. The emotional and physical toll was immeasurable, and the scars, both seen and unseen, are a constant reminder of the nightmare I endured. My journey, like so many others, is a testament to the profound impact of exploitation and the long, arduous path toward healing and reclaiming one's life.

My life had taken a turn for the worse. After being laid off from my job, I found myself struggling to secure another position. The job hunt was taking longer than I had hoped, and I was living week to week, my savings dwindling rapidly. Desperation crept in as I fell behind on my car payments and eventually lost my car. Soon after, I was evicted from the house I shared with a roommate due to unpaid rent. My life spiraled downward, each setback compounding the last.

One particularly grim evening, I stood in a WaWa convenience store, clutching the last $3.76 I had. I was contemplating what meager purchase I could make to sustain myself for just a bit longer. My mind was clouded with worry and despair. Then, out of nowhere, a man approached me. He remarked that I looked like I needed a friend and offered to pay for whatever I needed. In my vulnerable state, I thought, "how very kind," not realizing that this seemingly generous gesture was the first step into a world of unimaginable darkness.

I remember chatting with him that night. He had an easy charm, and his kindness felt like a lifeline in my sea of despair. He mentioned that he stopped at the WaWa every morning for a cup of coffee on his way to work. He said he would buy me breakfast if I was there around 10. Desperation and hunger drove me to be there waiting the next morning.

True to his word, he bought me breakfast. We chatted for about an hour, sitting comfortably in his car. He seemed genuinely interested in my situation, asking questions with a concerned and attentive demeanor. He was dressed in clean clothes, drove a nice car, and mentioned he had a family. He seemed respectable, a stark contrast to the chaotic mess my life had become.

After our conversation, he offered me a place to stay. It sounded like a miracle. I had nothing to lose at that point. That $3.76 was all I had left, and I had exhausted the generosity of my friends and family. My world had shrunk to a single, dire option. With no other avenues open, I accepted his offer, clinging to the hope that his kindness was genuine and that it might be a way to finally get back on my feet. Little did I know, this decision would lead me into an even darker and more treacherous place than I had ever imagined.

That was the beginning of the darkest, bleakest existence anyone could imagine. What initially seemed like a lifeline quickly unraveled into a nightmare. I had dabbled in drugs and alcohol in the past, but I was never an addict. These substances were luxuries I couldn't afford in my struggle to survive.

Once I moved in with him, everything changed. The kindness he initially showed vanished, replaced by manipulation and control. He introduced me to a world of drugs, using them as a tool to weaken my resolve and ensure my compliance. The substances that were once out of reach became readily available, and I found myself sinking deeper into dependency. It was a deliberate, calculated move on his part, stripping me of any remaining semblance of autonomy.

The abuse was relentless, both physical and psychological. I was coerced into activities I never imagined, trapped in a cycle of degradation and despair. Every aspect of my life was controlled by him, and I was isolated from any source of help or support. My identity, once a reflection of hope and dreams, disintegrated under the weight of exploitation and addiction. My existence became a blur of pain and survival, a far cry from the life I had once known.

Days blurred into years, each one indistinguishable from the next in the relentless grind of abuse and exploitation. I knew I had to get out, but the means of escape eluded me. I was trapped, ensnared by fear, addiction, and the manipulative grasp of my captor.

One day, fate intervened in an unexpected way: I was arrested for prostitution. I never imagined that this would be my path to salvation, but it was. Being locked in a jail cell, I was forcibly cut off from the drugs that had numbed my existence. Going through detox in that cold, sterile cell was absolutely horrible. The physical and emotional agony was beyond anything I had ever experienced. Every minute felt like an eternity, and I literally prayed that God would take me, so I wouldn't have to endure the pain for another second. It was the first time I had prayed in my life, a desperate plea from the depths of my suffering.

As the days of withdrawal dragged on, something remarkable happened. The fog began to lift, and a flicker of clarity and hope emerged. I realized that this arrest, this moment of utter despair, was also a turning point. In the sterile confines of that jail cell, I saw the possibility of a different life. It was the start of a long and arduous journey to reclaim my identity and rebuild my life from the shattered remnants of my past.

In jail, I met several other women who had experienced, and were experiencing, the same emotions and uncertainty. We were all bound by our shared stories of exploitation, addiction, and loss. Despite the bleakness of our situation, something remarkable began to happen. In our moments of vulnerability and pain, we started to cling to the one thing that offered a glimmer of hope: God.

We formed a small support group, sharing our stories, and encouraging each other to look beyond our current circumstances. Through tears and confessions, we found solace in each other's company and began to rediscover our faith. For many of us, it was the first time we had allowed ourselves to believe in something greater than our suffering.

We prayed together, finding strength in our collective voices and the hope that God could help us heal and guide us to a better future. In those prayer sessions, we found a sense of community and belonging that had been absent from our lives for so long. It was in this newfound faith that we began to see a path forward, one that led away from the darkness of our pasts and toward the possibility of redemption and recovery.

The jail cell, once a place of despair, became a space of transformation. We supported each other through the painful process of detox, sharing words of encouragement and faith. Slowly, the chains of our addictions and past traumas began to loosen. Together, we started to heal, piece by piece, guided by the belief that we were not alone and that a higher power was watching over us, giving us the strength to overcome our struggles.

Despite finding a sense of hope and community in jail, I still experienced moments of deep despair. The thought of rebuilding my life from scratch at age 44 was daunting. It wasn't just about piecing together fragments of my old life; it was about creating an entirely new one—a new support system, a new community, and a new identity. I had no idea where to start.

Each day presented a fresh set of challenges and fears. The comfort of the familiar, even when it was harmful, was gone. I had to navigate a world that had moved on without me, filled with people who had no understanding of the depths I had been to. I had to find housing, employment, and a way to stay sober—all without the safety nets that many take for granted.

My first steps were small and hesitant. Upon release, I connected with a local rehabilitation program that offered a lifeline of support. This program was a comprehensive resource, providing not just therapy and addiction counseling, but also practical support like job training, housing assistance, and life skills workshops. Each service was designed to help people like me regain their footing in a world that felt foreign and intimidating.

In this program, I began to build a new community. I met mentors who had dedicated their lives to helping others recover from trauma and addiction. These mentors were a wellspring of knowledge and empathy, guiding me with patience and understanding. They offered practical advice on navigating everyday challenges and emotional support when the weight of my past felt overwhelming.

I also met other survivors who had walked similar paths. These individuals became my allies and confidants, sharing their stories and listening to mine. We bonded over our shared experiences of pain and recovery, creating a network of support that was both healing and empowering. Together, we attended group therapy sessions where we could express our fears and hopes in a safe, non-judgmental environment.

Through job training programs, I learned new skills that opened up employment opportunities I had never considered before. The program provided mock interviews, résumé workshops, and even partnered with local businesses to help us find internships and job placements. This practical support was invaluable, giving me the tools and confidence to re-enter the workforce.

Housing assistance was another critical component of my recovery. The program helped me find a safe and stable place to live, far from the environments that had perpetuated my suffering. Having a secure home allowed me to focus on my recovery without the constant worry of where I would sleep each night.

Additionally, life skills workshops taught me how to manage finances, cook nutritious meals, and maintain a healthy lifestyle. These skills were essential for my independence and long-term success, helping me to build a foundation for a stable and fulfilling life.

As I immersed myself in this new community, I began to feel a sense of belonging and purpose that had been missing for so long. The connections I made and the skills I learned gradually replaced the fear and uncertainty with hope and determination. Each small step forward was a victory, a testament to my resilience and the support of those around me.

Rebuilding my life was an arduous journey, but with the guidance of the rehabilitation program and the support of my new community, I started to see a future where I could not only survive, but thrive. Each day brought new challenges and triumphs, and slowly, I began to reclaim my identity and my life.

Finding a faith-based support group was also pivotal. It was a place where I could continue to explore and deepen my faith, drawing strength from others who shared my belief in God's ability to heal and restore. These groups provided a sanctuary where I could speak openly about my struggles and receive the spiritual and emotional support I needed.

One of my greatest hurdles was learning to trust again—trusting myself to make better choices, trusting others to support me, and trusting in a future that seemed uncertain but hopeful. It was a slow, often painful process, marked by setbacks and triumphs. But with each passing day, I took one more step away from the darkness and closer to a life filled with purpose and possibility.

The journey was far from easy, but each day offered the opportunity for progress, no matter how small. Each step forward became a testament to my spirit's capacity for recovery and renewal. Through unwavering faith, steadfast support, and sheer determination, I began to build a life that was not just about survival, but about truly living.

With each passing day, I moved closer to a life filled with purpose and possibility. I embraced new experiences, cultivated healthy relationships, and pursued goals that once seemed out of reach. My days were no longer defined by fear and despair, but by the joy of discovering who I was and what I could achieve. My faith became an unwavering beacon, guiding me through the darkness and instilling a sense of purpose. This faith was not just in a higher power, but in myself and the inherent strength I discovered within.

This journey of rebuilding was about more than just putting the pieces of my life back together. It was about creating something entirely new—something stronger, more resilient, and filled with hope. It was about transforming from a state of mere existence into one of vibrant living, embracing the full spectrum of life's experiences with courage and grace.

Support from my new community played a pivotal role. Mentors offered wisdom and guidance, helping me navigate the complexities of my new life. Fellow survivors became a source of solidarity and strength, their shared experiences creating a bond that was both comforting and empowering. Through these connections, I found a network of care and encouragement that lifted me up during my toughest times.

Sheer determination drove me to push past my limits, to confront and overcome the obstacles that once seemed insurmountable. Each challenge I faced and conquered added to my resilience, building a foundation of confidence and self-worth. I pursued education and training, opening doors to opportunities I had never thought possible. I built new relationships based on trust and mutual respect, forming a support system that nurtured my growth and healing.

As I forged this new path, I learned to celebrate not just the major milestones, but the small victories as well. Every step forward, no matter how small, was a triumph over the past and a testament to my enduring spirit. For example, the first time I secured a job interview, it felt like a monumental achievement. I found joy in everyday moments, like savoring a homemade meal or completing a challenging task at work.

Reconnecting with my children was probably the hardest thing I did on this journey of rebuilding my life. Years of absence and pain had created a chasm between us, filled with unanswered questions and emotional wounds. Approaching them after such a long time was daunting, and I feared their rejection and the possibility that the damage was irreparable.

Our first meeting was laden with emotion. My heart pounded as I stood at their door, memories flooding back of the times I had missed—the birthdays, the milestones, the everyday moments that I had not been there to share. When the door opened, I saw the apprehension in their eyes, mirroring my own.

The initial conversations were strained, a mix of awkward silences, and tentative exchanges. I had to confront the guilt and shame of my past actions and the impact they had on my children. They, in turn, had to grapple with their feelings of abandonment and betrayal. We had a lot to unpack, and the process was neither quick nor easy.

We started with small steps. I made a point to be consistent, showing up when I said I would and being present in their lives as much as they would allow. Gradually, we began to rebuild trust. I shared my story with them, explaining the dark period of my life and the journey I was on to make things right. It was important for them to understand that I was committed to change and that my love for them had never wavered, even during the worst times.

We found common ground in simple activities. We cooked meals together, went for walks, and spent quiet evenings watching movies. These moments, though seemingly mundane, were incredibly healing. They allowed us to reconnect and rediscover each other outside the shadows of the past.

One of the most profound experiences was attending family therapy sessions. These sessions provided a safe space for all of us to express our feelings and work through our pain. It was in these sessions that I truly began to understand the depth of my children's hurt and the strength of their forgiveness.

Reconnecting with my children was a testament to the possibility of healing and redemption. It required patience, humility, and an unwavering commitment to making amends. The process was filled with tears and difficult conversations, but also with moments of profound joy and reconnection. Each step forward, no matter how small, reinforced the belief that, together, we could heal and build a future grounded in love and understanding.

This journey of rebuilding was a profound transformation, turning the fragmented pieces of my past into a mosaic of strength, resilience, and hope. Through incredible faith, unwavering support, and relentless determination, I crafted a life that was not just about survival, but about truly living—embracing each day with gratitude and optimism.

CHAPTER 8

Grind, Grit, and Glam

"Life ain't easy... never was, and still isn't."

When I was asked to share my story, the first thing I said was, "Life ain't easy... never was, and still isn't." I don't even know why I said it like that, but probably 'cause my whole life, I been feelin' like I'm just tryin' to survive. Growin' up in Newark, NJ, right in the middle of all that civil unrest, it was tough. Times was scary for Black folks back then. Every day felt like a battle just to make it through. We was out here fightin' for our rights, our lives, our dignity. It was rough, and it ain't like things magically got better overnight. So yeah, when I think back on it, it's no wonder I said, "life ain't easy. It never has been," and it seems like it never will be.

I knew at an early age I had to get outta Newark. There just wasn't any opportunity for me there. The streets was rough, and I saw too many folks around me get caught up in things that wasn't goin' nowhere. I didn't want to be a have-not; I wanted to do more, be more. I wanted to live without constantly worryin' 'bout how I was gonna exist day to day. I had dreams, and I knew stayin' in Newark would just keep me stuck in a cycle of struggle. I was determined to find a way out, to carve a path for myself where I could thrive, not just survive. I wanted a life where I could reach for somethin' better, where I could finally breathe without fear weighin' me down.

This is probably when I really started feelin' like life was gonna be harder for me than most. There were so few options for an uneducated young Black woman like me. Everywhere I turned, it seemed like doors were closin' before I even got close. Then one day, I looked across the river and saw NYC. That city felt like a whole different world, full of possibilities I couldn't even imagine back in Newark. I thought to myself, "Maybe that's my only option, my one shot at somethin' better." The Big Apple was callin' and I felt like maybe, just maybe, it could offer me a chance to break free from the struggle. It was scary, no doubt, but I knew if I stayed where I was, I'd just keep fightin' the same battles without ever winnin'. So, I set my sights on New York, hopin' it could be my way out, my chance to finally make somethin' of myself.

I had always liked fashion, so I decided to try my luck at Macy's. I figured if I could get my foot in the door there, maybe I could start buildin' somethin' better for myself. I had barely finished high school, but I knew I looked okay. I could dress sharp and carry myself with confidence, even if I didn't have much else goin' for me on paper. So, I walked into Macy's, hopin' they'd see somethin' in me, hopin' they'd give me a chance. The store was huge, bright, and full of all the latest trends. Just bein' there felt like I was a step closer to my dreams. I knew it wasn't gonna be easy, but I was determined to make it work. This was my shot, and I wasn't gonna let it slip away.

Macy's hired me, and I started in the shoe department. I won't say it was my dream job, but it helped me start building a dream. I was surrounded by stylish shoes and bustling crowds, and I quickly learned the ropes. Every day, I put on my best smile and helped customers find what they needed. It wasn't glamorous, but it was a start. I was finally earning my own money and gaining a sense of independence I hadn't felt before.

Working at Macy's gave me a taste of the fashion world, and I soaked up everything I could. I paid attention to trends, watched how the more experienced employees interacted with customers, and dreamed about where this job could eventually take me. It wasn't easy - long hours on my feet and dealing with all kinds of folks - but I held onto that dream. I knew that this was just the beginning. With every paycheck, I felt a little more hopeful, a little more determined to keep pushing forward and create a better future for myself.

I married, and we started a family. Yup, I was young, and the kids came fast, one after another. Life was a whirlwind of diapers, feedings, and sleepless nights. I don't know if I was truly happy or just doing what I thought I was supposed to do. It was a blur of responsibilities and routine, but I kept going because that's what you do.

I still worked as a clerk at Macy's, and while it wasn't glamorous, it brought in the money we needed to support the family. Every morning, I'd get up early, get the kids ready, and head off to work. The days were long and tiring, but seeing my children's faces at the end of the day made it worth it.

Balancing work and home was a constant juggle. I'd spend my days helping customers, always with a smile, and my nights taking care of the little ones. There wasn't much time for myself, but I found a strange sense of purpose in the chaos. Even though I sometimes wondered if I was just going through the motions, deep down, I knew I was doing it all for them—for my family.

It wasn't easy, but I learned to find joy in the small moments, like the way my baby would giggle or the pride I felt when I handed over my paycheck, knowing I was contributing to our future. Life wasn't perfect, but it was ours, and that made all the difference.

The years ran past me, blurring into a haze of memories and milestones. I don't know if I was running too—running from my past or running toward a new life. It all felt like a race, and I was just trying to keep up. Between raising kids, working long hours, and managing a household, I rarely had time to think, let alone consider if I was happy or content.

I had escaped Newark, that much was true. I had a life away from the chaos and fear that once surrounded me, but sometimes I wondered if I had truly found peace. My days were filled with routines and responsibilities, leavin' little room for thinkin' 'bout myself. It was all 'bout makin' ends meet, makin' sure my kids had a better future, and keepin' the wheels turnin'.

Lookin' back, it feels like I was on autopilot, movin' through life by sheer force of will. The kids grew up fast, each year bringin' new challenges and joys. My job at Macy's stayed steady, a constant source of income and stability. I took pride in my work, even if it wasn't what I had dreamed of as a child.

Every now and then, I'd catch a glimpse of my reflection in a store window and wonder 'bout the woman starin' back at me. Had I found what I was lookin' for? Had I built the life I wanted, or was I still searchin', still runnin'?

Despite the uncertainty, I knew one thing for sure: I had created a life far removed from the struggles of my youth. My family was safe, my kids were growin', and I had carved out a space for myself in a world that often seemed too big and too harsh. It wasn't perfect, but it was mine. And in those fleeting moments of quiet, I found a sense of accomplishment, and a flicker of hope for whatever lay ahead.

When the girls gathered to chat, we'd talk 'bout our lives and how we felt 'bout where we were. We'd sit around, sippin' on coffee or maybe somethin' a bit stronger, just tryna unwind from the day. Not one of them ever said they were "happy". They all said they were "just goin' through the motions of life."

We'd laugh and share stories, but underneath it all, there was this shared sense of struggle. Livin' wasn't easy, and it seemed like we were all just tryin' to make it through. Some of us had dreams we put on hold, some were dealin' with troubled marriages, and others were just plain tired from the constant grind.

We'd nod our heads in understanding, 'cause we were all in the same boat. The hustle, the sacrifices, the long hours at work, and then comin' home to more work. It was a lot, but we found comfort in each other, knowin' we weren't alone. We were all just doin' what we had to do, hopin' that one day things might get a little easier, a little brighter.

Talkin' with them helped me realize that even though we weren't livin' the lives we once dreamed of, we were survivin'. We were strong, and we were doin' the best we could with what we had. It wasn't perfect, but it was our reality, and we faced it together.

Then one day, it happened—my husband died unexpectedly. One day he was there, and the next, he was gone. We had three teenagers still at home, and my meager salary wasn't gonna cover all our bills. It felt like the ground had been snatched right out from under me.

Once again, I had to make a major decision. How was I gonna make more money to keep the household goin'? I was scared and overwhelmed at age 41, but I knew I had to keep pushin' forward for my kids. They needed me more than ever, and I couldn't let them down.

I started lookin' for extra work, anything that could bring in some more cash. I picked up extra shifts at Macy's, workin' late into the night and on weekends. I also started doin' hair on the side, somethin' I was pretty good at from way back. Word got around the neighborhood, and soon I had folks comin' to me for braids, weaves, and perms.

It wasn't easy. There were nights I barely slept, worryin' 'bout how we was gonna make it through the month, but I kept goin' and kept hustlin'. I knew I had no other choice. The kids needed food, clothes, and a roof over their heads and I was determined to give it to them.

Every dollar I made went straight to the bills, takin' care of my people. We tightened up, cut out all the extras, made do with what we had.

Times was rough, no doubt, but we got through. Little by little, we found our groove, figured out how to make it work.

I stretched them paychecks like they was rubber bands, makin' sure every penny counted. When it came time to shop, it was all about needs, not wants. And if somethin' unexpected popped up—a doctor bill, somethin' broke down—we got real creative. We fixed things ourselves, traded favors with folks, even sold off stuff that was just takin' up space.

Them small wins? We learned to celebrate 'em. A good home-cooked meal felt special, like love was cooked right in. Workin' together out in the yard on a Saturday, that was our kind of family time. We laughed more over the little things, like patchin' up clothes instead of buyin' new, or findin' a good deal on somethin' we needed. We stuck close, leaned on each other, and found joy in the simple stuff. Every cutback, every sacrifice, it was like layin' one more brick on our path forward. And even when money was tight, we felt rich in ways you can't count.

Through it all, I realized just how strong I was. Life kept throwin' curveballs, but I kept swingin'. I did what I had to do to keep my family afloat, and even though it was hard, I knew we would make it through.

"Yup, I was able to get outta Newark and survive!" I say, shaking my head at the memories. "It ain't been easy, but I made it. I hustled hard, worked every shift I could, saved every dime. At night, I did my friends' hair—balancing those with my daytime jobs. Any free time I had, I spent telling folks about my hair business."

I lean in, emphasizing the grind. "I networked like crazy, you know? Handing out flyers, offering free services just to get my name out there. I wasn't shy. I knew I had to make it happen."

A small smile spreads across my face as I remember the early hustle. "I even rented a chair at a local shop for a while. Learned the ropes, built my client base. Slowly but surely, I started to get steady customers. You know how it is—word gets around."

I cut back on unnecessary expenses, got a small loan, and put everything into securing my own space. I did my own renovations, found good deals on equipment, and put together a welcoming vibe with a personal touch. Today, I have my own salon. No more shifts at Macy's—I've got my own place, filled with steady clients. The space is small, but it's mine, and it's always buzzing with laughter, gossip, and the hum of hair dryers. Folks come in, I make 'em look good, and they leave feelin' even better. Every step was tough, but the grind was worth it.

I built this business from the ground up, with hard work and determination and my regulars come back 'cause they know I have skills and a big heart. I love seein' their smiles when they look in the mirror. Every style, every cut, every braid is a testament to the journey I've been on.

At the end of the day, I think 'bout all those years, all those struggles, and it hits me just how far I've come. I smile to myself, knowin' I was able to push through the hard stuff and today, I ain't just survivin' no more, I'm thrivin'! I got outta Newark, built a life for my kids, and now I'm livin' my dream! It's a good feelin', knowin' I made it through, stronger and wiser. Life ain't perfect, but it's mine, and I'm proud of every step I took to get here.

I sit back, crossing my arms with a sense of pride. "That's how I did it. No shortcuts, just straight-up grind."

Section 4 Introduction - Thankful

As they acknowledged the necessity for change, these women found the courage to take incremental steps toward their new goals. They sought out new experiences, learned new skills, and connected with supportive communities that nurtured their growth.

The journey was often challenging and required a deep commitment to personal development, but it was also deeply rewarding. Each small victory reinforced their belief in their ability to shape their own destinies.

Many did not tread this path alone and invited entrusted mentors and friends to offer wisdom and guidance as they navigated through their journey. This support helped them tap into their innermost thoughts and feelings, helping them gain clarity on what truly mattered to them. They explored their passions, values, and deepest desires, and what they uncovered was the path to a more fulfilling existence. One that was special to them.

Moreover, they embraced a proactive attitude, seeking solutions rather than dwelling on problems. They actively sought feedback, adapted their strategies, and remained open to new ideas and perspectives. This adaptability was crucial in navigating the unpredictable nature of their journeys. By maintaining a flexible approach, they could pivot and adjust their plans as needed, ensuring that temporary setbacks did not derail their overall progress.

The transformation experienced by these women serves as a testament to the resilience of the human spirit. Taking proactive steps and seeking out supportive communities demonstrated that change is possible at any stage of life. Their stories encourage us to look beyond our immediate circumstances and to trust in our ability to shape our destinies. As we read about their journeys, we are reminded that redefining our lives and pursuing our deepest aspirations is never too late. Through their courage and determination, these women not only transformed their lives, but also paved the way for others to follow in their footsteps, proving that pursuing fulfillment and joy is a journey worth embarking upon.

So, for all the women out there seeking their dreams, let us embrace the discomfort, lean into the unknown, and trust that the journey is worth the destination. It is only by daring to dream and by daring to act that we can truly create the life of our dreams.

CHAPTER 9

The Other Side of Perfect

"In the vibrant smiles of the Red Hatters, I discovered that true beauty lies not in youth, but in the joy of living fully and embracing the passage of time with grace."

In my twenties, I serendipitously came across the enchanting world of the "Red Hatters" club. The memory still lingers vividly in my mind - those older ladies gathered at lunch, sporting striking red and purple hats that seemed to radiate with a vibrancy that was infectious. Their demeanor was a sight to behold, exuding happiness and confidence, proudly displaying genuine smiles that sparkled in their eyes along with their festive attire. At that moment, I couldn't help but perceive them as somewhat antiquated, out of touch with the fast-evolving times. Little did I know, however, that it was not them who were out of step, but rather I who had yet to grasp the timeless wisdom and spirit of living joyfully and contently in the present. It would be years later, as life unfolded its lessons, that I would come to appreciate the beauty and significance of their exuberance and camaraderie within the "Red Hatters" community.

As the last decade unfolded, I found myself face to face with a reflection in the mirror that bore a striking resemblance to one of those radiant older women from the "Red Hatters" club. Initially, I almost mistook her for a visiting family member, assuming I could simply send her on her way by masking her presence with hair color, foundation to conceal wrinkles, and spandex to tame my waistline. Yet, despite my efforts to alter my physical appearance, she remained, steadfastly gazing back at me from the mirror. A poignant reminder of the passage of time and the inevitable march of aging.

As I gazed into the mirror, studying the reflection that stared back at me with a mix of familiarity and intrigue, I couldn't help but notice a subtle change in the essence of the image before me. Amidst the lines etched by time and the nuances of expression that told stories of laughter and contemplation, there was a flicker of a spark that seemed to have dulled over the years. It was as if the eyes held secrets untold, yearning for a touch of vibrancy and a whisper of excitement that had faded into the background of daily routines and responsibilities.

The laugh lines around the corners of my eyes, once etched with the joy of shared moments and heartfelt connections, now seemed to murmur of a deeper longing, a yearning for "the more" that eluded clear definition. I found myself wondering, "What was it that stirred within her," prompting this quiet yet persistent restlessness that lingered beneath the surface of contentment. Was it a craving for more meaningful connections, a thirst for knowledge found within the pages of captivating books, or perhaps a desire for shared moments of laughter and conversation over leisurely lunches with kindred spirits?

From an external perspective, it appeared that I had everything one could desire—a strong and loving marriage, a close-knit community of supportive friends, a cherished family, and a successful career marked by achievements and accolades. Despite these outward markers of fulfillment and accomplishment, there lingered persistent whispers in the depths of my being, echoing the haunting question: "Is this all there is?"

Maybe it was living the Instagram-worthy life, while secretly craving a deeper connection with the universe! It's like trying to sip champagne with a straw - feeling like you're missing out on the bubbles. My current facade was kept together with wrinkle cream and spandex like a superhero costume for the middle-aged.

I mean, here I was, juggling relationships, accomplishments, and stability like a pro, but deep down there was this little voice in my head going, "Hey, there's gotta be more to life than just collecting achievements and perfecting my bridge game." It was like my soul was on a treasure hunt and all it found was a bunch of material stuff and a slightly deflated ego.

I had retired just a few months ago and everyone kept asking me, "Aren't you thrilled to be rid of deadlines, office small talk, and the dreaded morning alarm?" Honestly, I was hesitant to admit that, no, I wasn't exactly thrilled to fade into the sunset just yet. I felt that was what my future held for me as I had lunch dates, played mahjong, and tried new dinner recipes.

So, there I was, caught in this epic battle between gratitude for my blessings and a relentless craving for that elusive "more." It was like trying to choose between a cozy Netflix binge and a spontaneous adventure – both tempting, but one had way more potential for personal growth and mosquito bites. Thus, my quest for a soul-stirring, authentic existence began, armed with nothing but a sprinkle of fear and a whole lot of determination.

Hindsight really is like wearing a pair of glasses with perfect vision. As I reflected on my past while pondering my next adventure, it became painfully clear that signs had been popping up for years, waving at me like overenthusiastic traffic cops. It wasn't just the wrinkles staring back at me in the mirror; it was the gut feelings I'd been brushing aside like crumbs off a table, convincing myself I was just tired and needed a recharge. Thoughts of vacations spent by the pool or beach surfaced often, but I never made a move to do it. Little did I know, those feelings were trying to tell me I needed more than just a power nap on a beach towel to reboot my life.

It's a classic conundrum: finally having the time to chase adventures in your golden years, yet feeling like you're tiptoeing through a minefield when it comes to dropping the bombshell on your spouse that you want more out of life. For ages, my husband and I fantasized about those carefree days by the pool, sipping on those oh-so-tempting vacation beverages. I found myself disillusioned; this wasn't the life of leisure I imagined, sipping piña coladas while waves serenade the shore. It dawned on me: I couldn't bear the thought of endless dinner parties and retelling the same old stories. I craved fresh tales, adventures untold. New stories, new places, and some new faces.

The real fun kicked off the moment I mustered the courage to declare, "I want more!" I wasn't ready to hit the brakes on expanding my mind or stretching my comfort zone. I decided to finally shake things up and dive headfirst into the great unknown, surprising not just my husband, but maybe even myself! No expectations, just the sheer thrill of trying something completely different.

No more dealing with employees, rigid schedules, pesky deadlines, or feeling obligated to be a retiree. The possibilities were as vast as a buffet of adventures waiting to be devoured. Who would've thought that by saying "No" to certain things, I was actually saying "Yes" to a world brimming with exciting possibilities? It was time to embrace the unexpected and groove to the beat of my own unique journey.

I had an eclectic mishmash on my "to try" list: floral arranging, surfing, pasta making, mahjong, nantucket basket weaving, and jewelry making. Talk about a grab bag of activities! It's like my bucket list went on a blind date with a random assortment of interests. But, if these are the final chapters of my book of life, I might as well throw caution to the wind and give whatever strikes my fancy a shot, right? Who knows, maybe I'll end up being the Michelangelo of sourdough bread or the Steve Jobs of water aerobics. I will spoil the story now by letting you know I was not a star at either of those things, but I discovered that the possibilities were as endless as they are delightfully unpredictable.

Some of my friends thought I was starting to lose my marbles, but little did they know, I was actually beginning to find them! Sure, there were a few false starts along the way – like my ill-fated attempt at flower arranging. I figured it was a simple way to dip my toes into the waters of expanding my horizons. I mean, who doesn't love fresh flowers brightening up their home? I thought I had inherited my mother's knack for floral artistry, but the moment the instructor unveiled our project, I knew I was in trouble. It was like she was handing me a paintbrush and expecting me to recreate the Mona Lisa! Let's just say, I quickly realized my mom's green thumb skipped over me entirely.

Picture this: a room full of hopeful students clutching their flowers and me, standing there with my arrangement looking like a hedgehog that had a run-in with a lawnmower, while others were crafting masterpieces worthy of magazine covers. My creation looked more like a botanical Frankenstein. The instructor, bless her heart, tried her best to encourage me behind a strained smile. By the end of the class, my bouquet had wilted along with my hopes of becoming a floral Picasso.

That flower arranging fiasco may not have blossomed into a hidden talent, but at least I stretched my comfort zone like a champion contortionist! I leaned in, alright – leaned in and discovered exactly where my boundaries lay. Instead of sulking over my lack of floral finesse, I proudly checked it off my list of potential talents. And you know what? Although I didn't bloom into a floral Picasso, I reached out for something different, and that's worth celebrating.

My mishmash of interests had friends scratching their heads, my husband giving me quizzical looks, and me? Well, I was blossoming like a garden in springtime. I dived into every single item on that list, and while some were more "one-night stand" than "lasting love." Turns out the spark I thought I was losing was just waiting for the right moment to explode into a blazing inferno of curiosity and self-discovery.

Throughout my life journey, I've come to recognize a recurring pattern: the tendency to categorize friends as if they were mere items on a shopping list. "She's the culinary genius, she's the altruist, she's the entrepreneurial whiz," and so forth. These labels seem to cling to individuals with a tenacity akin to glitter stubbornly adhering after a crafting session. Intrigued by this phenomenon, I resolved to amass labels like prized limited edition stickers. After all, don't these distinctions render individuals captivating? Yet, beneath these surface labels lie depths waiting to be explored and complexities yearning to be understood. So, while labels may offer a glimpse into someone's character, they are but a fraction of the rich tapestry that makes each person truly fascinating.

So, armed with my hodgepodge of interests and a dash of rebellious spirit, I set out on a mission to accumulate as many labels as I could. Forget being pigeonholed into just one category – I was determined to be the jack-of-all-trades, the Renaissance woman of our friend group. From mastering the art of gourmet cooking to organizing charity events, and from delving into the intricacies of business strategy to exploring the depths of philosophical thought, I embraced every opportunity to expand my repertoire. After all, life's too short to be boxed in by labels, especially when there are so many adventures waiting to be had! Each label I collected was not just a badge of honor, but a testament to the diverse experiences and passions that shaped my journey. With each new label, I found myself growing, evolving, and uncovering new facets of my identity that defied conventional categorization.

Sure, I still had those pesky worries about what my friends might be whispering behind my back, but with each new adventure, my confidence grew stronger, drowning out the noise of their doubts. It was as if every step I took into the unknown fortified my spirit, silencing the faint murmurs of skepticism that lingered in the air.

With newfound confidence bubbling within me, I began to approach life with a sense of exhilaration I hadn't felt before. There was an undeniable shift in my mindset—a spark that made me believe that the only true downside to trying something new was the investment of my time and resources. But even that seemed like a small price to pay when weighed against the potential rewards. Every unknown became a canvas waiting for me to make my mark, every untraveled path an open invitation to explore. The usual hesitations, those nagging doubts that had once held me back, faded into the background, replaced by a bold, almost reckless curiosity.

I had grown tired of the comfort zone, the predictable rhythms of daily life that offered little more than safety. The idea of remaining static, of living in a world of "what ifs" and "maybes," no longer held any appeal. Instead, I began to see every new opportunity—whether it was a chance to travel, to learn a new skill, or to embark on a creative venture—as a thrilling adventure in and of itself. The risks no longer felt daunting; they were exciting. The prospect of failure, once a source of anxiety, now became a minor blip on the radar of progress. If anything, failure was simply another experience to learn from, another stepping stone toward something greater.

I recall one particular moment when this shift became most apparent. I had been invited to a conference halfway across the country—an event where I knew no one and had no real ties to the subject matter, but I felt a strong pull to attend. Without overthinking it, I booked the ticket, packed my bags, and stepped into the unknown. In the past, I would have second-guessed myself, worrying about whether it was worth the time, the money, the effort. But this time, I felt a quiet thrill in the spontaneity. I arrived at the event alone, unsure of what to expect, but with an openness that made me see every conversation as a possibility. What followed was a weekend full of serendipitous encounters. I met people who shared my interests, discovered new ideas that sparked my creativity, and found connections that would later turn into collaborations.

In retrospect, it seemed so simple—just an impulsive decision to go to a place I had never been, to a room full of strangers. But in that space, surrounded by new faces and fresh perspectives, I realized how much growth had occurred in such a short time. It wasn't just about what I had gained in terms of tangible outcomes—though there were plenty of those—it was the internal shift I had undergone. I saw how much my world had expanded by stepping out of my comfort zone and allowing myself to simply *be* in a new, unfamiliar space. The investment of time and money seemed minuscule compared to the wealth of experiences I had gained.

This sense of possibility seeped into every corner of my life. Suddenly, the idea of trying something new—whether it was starting a project, pursuing a new hobby, or taking on a new challenge—wasn't a source of anxiety, but of excitement. I embraced risk not as something to be feared, but as an opportunity for personal growth and exploration. The unfamiliar no longer felt like a threat but a doorway to something greater, and I no longer hesitated to walk through it.

Each new risk I took added to the confidence I had started to cultivate, creating a cycle of boldness and discovery. I learned to trust that no matter where the path led, I would be better for having walked it. The world, once full of obstacles, now felt brimming with possibility. And the best part? I began to realize that the only true limits I faced were the ones I set for myself. So long as I kept pushing past those boundaries, there would always be something new to discover, some new challenge to tackle, and some new part of myself to uncover.

The risks weren't just opportunities for success—they were opportunities for transformation. With every leap of faith, I felt more alive, more capable, and more connected to the ever-expanding horizon in front of me. The beauty of it all was that the journey itself—the willingness to take the step, to embrace the unknown—became as meaningful as the destination. And that belief, that every risk was simply a chance to grow, kept me moving forward with purpose, curiosity, and an open heart.

With every new trial and tribulation came a treasure trove of stories, ripe for sharing at every opportunity. While the tribulations may have felt like stumbling blocks at the time, they ended up being my best anecdotes. It wasn't just the stories that enriched my life – it was the connections I forged along the way. They're the threads that weave together the chapters of my life, crafting a story so exciting, I don't want to stop.

That persistent murmur, incessantly questioning, "Is this all there is?" — it's vanished, replaced by a serene contentment. It may not resemble the grand prize I once chased fervently, but it's precisely what my soul craved. I yearned to stretch my boundaries, to explore uncharted territories, to uncover hidden depths within myself. In my quest to reach those goals, I've stumbled upon a profound sense of fulfillment, a treasure more precious than any skill or talent I could have amassed.

I may not be wearing the bold hats I once scoffed at in my twenties, but guess what? I'm having just as much fun as those ladies who sported them back then. Life has taught me that the real joy isn't in the hat's color or style, but rather in discovering the "more" that brings the sparkle back to the eyes and fills the laugh lines with genuine joy.

In embracing this truth, I've found a profound liberation from the shackles of societal expectations and the relentless pressure to conform to a predetermined image or trend. Instead, I dance freely in the expansive realm of self-expression, relishing the opportunity to explore every facet of my identity, and pursue passions and dreams that harmonize with the essence of my being.

As I navigate this journey of self-discovery, my wardrobe may undergo transformations, but the fervor for life blazes within me, radiating each day with a vibrant tapestry of adventure and possibility. With each step forward, I am propelled by the realization that true happiness transcends the superficial layers of outward appearance. It thrives in the rich soil of authenticity and blossoms through the connections we cultivate along our shared path of growth and understanding.

CHAPTER 10

Beyond Burnout: Reigniting the Spark

"It dawned on me that patching up problems wasn't the same as solving them. The real work was digging out the roots, and that required a willingness to get down and dirty to confront the mess head-on."

Growing up in the 70s, I was a curious child, always eager to explore the world around me. My neighborhood was a charming enclave of bustling shops, cozy bookstores, and friendly faces. The streets were alive with energy, and every corner seemed to hold a new discovery. It was a time when children roamed freely, and the neighborhood moms, including mine, encouraged us to spend as much time outside as possible. Whether I was riding my bike down quiet streets or peeking into shop windows, my days were filled with wonder. Even at the tender age of five or six, I was a regular explorer.

Though I rarely had money, I never felt deprived. Occasionally, my grandfather would slip me some change, and with great excitement, I'd head straight for the pharmacy down the street. I'd hop onto a stool at the restaurant counter, sipping on a cherry coke, savoring every bubble and sweetness. Ice cream was a rare treat, so I usually settled for soda or a piece of bubble gum. Afterward, I'd wander through the aisles, fascinated by the makeup displays and the countless drugstore items, wondering who bought them and why. This curiosity was insatiable. Why did people buy certain things? What were they for? Who would use them? My mind buzzed with questions I wasn't always sure how to answer.

Soon, my explorations led me to the library. I would bombard my mom, grandmother, and aunts with questions, but there were certain topics, especially for a young girl, that were off-limits. Determined to find answers, I'd hop back on my bike and pedal to the public library, spending hours devouring books on subjects that fascinated me. I was equally a fixture at the school library, checking out books during breaks and pestering my teachers with questions.

One evening, I remember watching my aunt as she typed up work reports. I was mesmerized by the rhythmic clacking of the keys and begged her to teach me. We had an old typewriter my dad had found and set up in our home. After some thought, he bought an ink ribbon for it, and my aunt sat down with me to teach the basics. I was only eleven, but my years of piano lessons had made my fingers nimble and strong. Before long, I was typing at an impressive speed of 100 words per minute. Learning to type felt like my first real step into the adult world— a skill that would serve me well in the business realm for decades to come. My dad and grandfather both recognized this relentless drive to learn. They ran the family business and taught me the ABC's of business throughout my teenage years as well as prodding me to take business courses in high school and college to round out my business knowledge.

Reflecting on those early years, I see how the countless hours of wandering the neighborhood, fueled by curiosity, led me on a lifelong journey of discovery. Every book, every question, every moment of exploration were all stepping stones, shaping the path that would guide me into the future.

In my 40s, I felt a yearning for change. I had been immersed in the business world for so long that it felt like second nature, yet something no longer fit. I was restless, waking up each morning with a vague sense of dissatisfaction, even though by all measures, I had "made it." My career was solid, my family was thriving, and life had settled into a predictable, almost comforting routine. Yet, I felt an unsettling ache, as though something crucial was missing.

It wasn't just the school schedules that had become more hectic with my children's activities, it was something more internal. The tipping point came one day in a moment I still replay in my mind. I was sitting at a business meeting with a client I'd been working with for years. We had just finished going over yet another quarterly review of sales projections. The meeting went well enough, but something about it felt different this time. As I sat there listening to the same old jargon about market shares and customer retention, I caught a glimpse of my reflection in the glass conference table. Was this what I wanted to be doing for the rest of my life?

That night, I came home later than usual. The kids were already in bed, and my husband was sitting on the couch watching sports. I could feel the familiar exhaustion settling in, but beneath it, there was a quiet, insistent whisper. "Is this it?"

I poured myself a glass of wine and sat down next to him. He looked over from the TV and he could tell something was off. "You okay?" he asked, muting the TV.

"I'm not sure," I admitted, staring into my cup. "I'm just... I don't know if I can keep doing this. It's the same problems over and over, and it's starting to feel meaningless."

He was silent for a moment, then said, "Maybe that's your sign. Maybe it's time to do something else."

His words stuck with me. I replayed that conversation in my head for days, feeling torn between the security of what I knew and the yearning for something new. It was easier said than done, though. How do you walk away from something you've built your entire life around? I wasn't even sure what that "something else" looked like yet.

My transition to consulting was gradual, but even as I took on small projects, I started noticing a pattern that made me feel increasingly uneasy. Every business I worked with had the same surface-level problems—low sales, poor marketing strategies, disorganized management—but underneath, there was always a deeper, human element. The owners and employees were overwhelmed, burned out, or stuck in cycles of negative thinking. I remember one particular client, a family-run business I'd been consulting for a year.

Sitting across from me was the daughter of the founder, visibly frustrated. Her father had handed the reins to her a few years ago, but the company was floundering. We were in the middle of reviewing operational procedures, but it was clear that wasn't the real issue.

"I just don't get it," she said, exasperated, running her hands through her hair. "We've tried everything—new marketing strategies, training programs, cutting costs. Why isn't anything working?"

I could see the exhaustion in her eyes. She had inherited not just a business, but the weight of family expectations. I paused for a moment before responding. "Marla," I said gently, "what's really going on here? I'm not asking about the business. I mean, how are you feeling about all of this?"

She stared at me, taken aback by the shift in the conversation, but then she let out a long sigh. "Honestly? I'm completely overwhelmed. I feel like I'm failing my family. No matter what I do, it's never enough. I don't even know if this is what I want anymore."

That was the moment I realized that fixing surface-level problems wasn't enough. If I didn't address the human side of business—the fears, insecurities, and emotional weight people carried—I was only pulling out weeds that would grow back. The root of the problem was always deeper, tangled in emotions and personal history.

It reminded me of gardening, something I did to clear my mind. Pulling weeds was a temporary solution, but if you didn't dig out the root, they'd always return. Business was the same. I could create the best strategies in the world, but if the people running the business weren't okay, neither was the business.

A specific event, however, pushed me to truly confront this idea. It was during a meeting with another client, a startup owner who was juggling everything from product development to customer service. We were supposed to discuss her marketing plan, but she was visibly distracted.

"Sorry," she said, apologizing for the third time as she glanced at her phone. "I'm just so... stressed. I can't focus. My son's been having issues at school, and I'm trying to hold everything together. Honestly, I don't know how much longer I can do this."

Something about her words struck me hard. It was the same look I had seen in my own reflection, the same exhaustion, the same question of "Is this it?"

As I left that meeting, I realized I didn't want to just help businesses anymore. I wanted to help women who were driven but weighed down by the pressures of business and life. I wanted to help them dig out their roots, clear the emotional clutter, and truly thrive—not just survive in their ventures.

That's when life coaching found me. At first, I dismissed it. I wasn't sure if I wanted to go through all the certifications required. But the more I researched, the more it made sense. Life coaching was about helping people tackle the personal blocks that held them back, and those blocks were often the root cause of business problems. The more I studied, the more it resonated with me. This was the missing piece, the link between my love for solving business challenges and my desire to help people on a deeper level.

I began life coaching with a small group of women, all eager to start their own businesses but held back by self-doubt. I remember my first client who was hesitant to even call herself an entrepreneur. "I'm not like those women who just... go for it," she admitted during our first session. "I don't know if I have what it takes."

We spent weeks unraveling her fears, talking through her insecurities. Slowly, she began to shift her mindset. I could see the change in her posture, her energy, her confidence. When she finally launched her first business, the joy in her voice when she called to tell me was contagious. "I did it!" she said, breathless with excitement. "I actually did it!"

Moments like that were why I knew I had made the right decision. Life coaching wasn't just about business advice—it was about transformation, about empowering women to see their own potential and step into their power.

As I embraced life coaching, another passion stirred within me: writing. I had always been an avid journaler, but now, I felt a pull to share my story and insights with others. The shelves of journals I had filled over the years began to beckon me. I realized that everything I had learned—the business lessons, the personal struggles, the triumphs of my clients—was a story worth telling.

So, here I am, once again at the brink of a new chapter, ready to share what I've experienced in hopes that others will find their own lightbulb moments, dig deep into their own roots, and plant the seeds for their own success.

Conclusion

The stories you've read share common threads and themes that resonate deeply and universally. All over 40, each woman found herself at a significant crossroads, feeling an urgent need to shift her narrative. They had reached a point in their lives best described as paused, a state often precipitated by profound life changes such as divorce, the death of a loved one, or significant career upheavals. These pauses were not mere momentary lulls, but were deeply entrenched in the habit of looking back at their pasts with regret or down at their current circumstances with a sense of despair. This backward and downward focus was a substantial factor contributing to their stagnation.

For many, this shift wasn't instantaneous. It required vulnerability and self-compassion, allowing themselves the grace to recognize their own strength in the face of uncertainty. Some found solace in creative pursuits, others in reconnecting with lost passions or forging new relationships. And while the past still held its weight, they began to see it not as a source of limitation, but as a foundation from which they could build something new. Slowly, they learned to stop measuring their worth against what they hadn't done or what had been lost, and instead began to focus on the untapped potential within them. What had once been a period of pause transformed into a fertile ground for reinvention—a realization that they could still shape their futures with purpose, courage, and joy. The crossroads were no longer places of stagnation but stepping stones toward the lives they were still meant to live.

For example, the stories of women who spoke of their experiences dealing with tumultuous divorces. They found themselves constantly ruminating on years they felt had been wasted in unhappy marriages. Every morning, they would wake up with a heavy heart, their minds replaying past mistakes and missed opportunities. This relentless focus on the past trapped them in a cycle of regret and sorrow - their pain blinding them from the opportunities that laid in front of them.

Similar parallels can be drawn with the woman who sold her business. The change in responsibilities left her feeling lost and purposeless, her days filled with restlessness. Eventually, she could only focus on her perceived shortcomings and the uncertainty of her current situation, which only deepened her despair and hindered her ability to move forward.

Our 52-year-old widow faced a different kind of loss. After her husband's sudden death, she felt completely lost and isolated. Once filled with love and laughter, her home now echoed with silence and sorrow. The grief she felt was overwhelming and she struggled to find meaning and direction in a world that had been irrevocably changed. Her days were marked by an unrelenting sense of emptiness and longing for the past.

However, each woman experienced a pivotal moment when she decided to shift her narrative. This shift was not just a change in their stories, but a profound transformation in how they perceived their lives. By consciously redirecting their focus from what was behind them - or beneath them - they began to look forward and outward, ready to embrace new possibilities and opportunities. This transformative shift in perspective allowed them to break free from the confines of their paused states.

Transformative shifts like the one our human trafficking survivor went through which allowed her to find a local support group for women who had experienced similar struggles. Through sharing her story and hearing others', she began to see that her past did not define her. She started focusing on what she wanted to achieve in the future, setting small, manageable goals that gradually reignited her sense of purpose. This change in perspective even encouraged her to participate in painting classes, something she had always wanted to do, but never had the courage to pursue. The act of creating art became a therapeutic outlet, filling her life with color and joy.

Another woman wrote about how she found solace in volunteering at a community center. She discovered that helping others allowed her to shift her attention from her own troubles to the needs of those around her. This outward focus brought her a sense of fulfillment and opened doors to new career opportunities. She discovered a passion for teaching and eventually transitioned into a role as an educator, finding a renewed sense of purpose and satisfaction.

A grief counseling group was the turning point for a woman dealing with her husband's passing. There, she met others who had experienced similar losses, and their shared experiences provided comfort and understanding. She also took up gardening, a hobby she and her husband had enjoyed together. Tending to her garden became a way to honor his memory and find peace. Over time, the garden blossomed, much like her renewed spirit.

Each story exemplifies the transformative power of shifting our focus from past and present despair to future possibilities and outward connections. Through these changes, the women in these stories redefined their identities and created meaningful, joyful lives, demonstrating that no matter the age or circumstance, a brighter, more fulfilling future is always within reach. Their journeys are a testament to the power of narrative change, illustrating how altering one's perspective can lead to profound personal growth and a more vibrant, hopeful future.

So, the question we have to ask you is this: what was it about the title and cover of this book that caught your attention? Are you currently feeling like your life is on pause, stuck in a rut, or trapped in a cycle of monotony? Perhaps you're feeling restless, discontented, or unfulfilled with where you are right now. Are you yearning for a change, a fresh start, or a way to shift your narrative to something more meaningful and satisfying? This book might just hold the key to unlocking the transformation you're seeking.

None of the stories told on these pages include a magical ingredient for transforming from restlessness to contentment, but all these women have made profound changes later in life. They have taken control of their destinies, reshaping their paths through resilience, courage, and determination. Each narrative is a testament to the power of self-reflection, personal growth, and the unwavering belief in the possibility of a brighter future. These women have faced their struggles head-on, navigated through their darkest moments, and emerged stronger and more empowered. Their journeys illustrate that while there is no quick fix or enchanted solution, real and lasting transformation is achievable through intentional action and the willingness to embrace change.

The stories told in this book were written with the intent to let others know that they are not alone in their journeys. While everyone's path is unique, we all share similar emotions, challenges, and triumphs. By delving into the experiences of others, we find comfort and solidarity, realizing that our struggles are not isolated. These narratives serve as a mirror reflecting the universal aspects of the human experience. Through reading and hearing about someone else's battles and victories we often find that our own burdens become more manageable.

Our goal in writing this book is that these stories provide hope, inspiration, and practical insights, demonstrating that despite our present difficulties, it is possible to cope, adapt, and make the necessary changes to transform our lives. We hope we have inspired each of you to shift your narrative and see that the path to a more fulfilling and meaningful life is always within reach. Always waiting for you to take the first step.

Anita Comisky

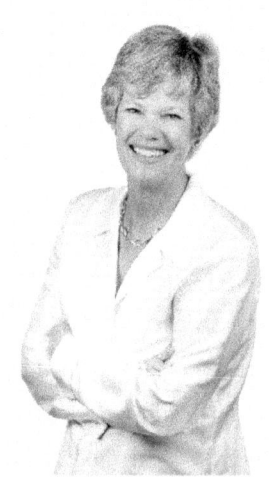

Background: An indomitable force of creativity and enterprise, Anita embodies the spirit of a true Renaissance woman, having embarked on a multifaceted journey that has taken her from the graceful courts of tennis to the enchanting world of artisanal confections and the dynamic realm of startup finance. Her life story is a tapestry woven with threads of passion, innovation, and unwavering determination.

🐾 **Transition to Candy Making:** With a zest for exploration and a palate for the extraordinary, Anita delved into the art of candy making with an artisanal flair that set her creations apart in a sea of sweetness. From handcrafted toffee infused with exotic flavors to selling live from her own kitchen on HSN that sparked joy in the hearts of all who beheld them, her confections became a culinary symphony of taste, texture, and imagination. This philanthropic twist added a deeper layer of purpose and meaning to Anita's culinary legacy, transforming her sweet treats into agents of empowerment and opportunity for those in need.

Anita's story is a testament to the transformative power of entrepreneurship infused with compassion and a commitment to giving back to the community. Through her delicious creations and her dedication to supporting women on their journey to a better future, Anita has not only left a lasting impact on the world of confectionery but also on the lives of those she touches with her generosity and kindness.

💼 **Entrepreneurial Journey:** Embracing the challenges and opportunities of the startup landscape, Anita brought her unique blend of creativity and analytical acumen to the forefront as a bean counter par excellence. With a sharp mind for strategy, a meticulous attention to detail, and a knack for financial foresight, she became a trusted advisor to budding entrepreneurs and seasoned business owners alike, guiding them through the intricacies of budgeting, forecasting, and financial planning with poise and precision.

🚀 **Innovative Spirit:** Fueled by an insatiable thirst for innovation and a bold vision for the future, Anita continues to push the boundaries of what is possible, constantly seeking new horizons to conquer and new challenges to overcome. Her pioneering spirit serves as a beacon of inspiration for those around her, encouraging them to embrace change, embrace risk, and embrace the transformative power of entrepreneurship as a force for positive change in the world.

🔥 **Legacy of Empowerment:** As she reflects on the chapters of her storied career and looks ahead to the adventures yet to come, Anita leaves a legacy of empowerment, resilience, and unyielding passion for the pursuit of excellence. Her journey is a testament to the boundless potential that lies within each of us to shape our destinies, defy expectations, and leave an indelible mark on the world through the sheer force of our creativity and determination.

Michelle Belloit

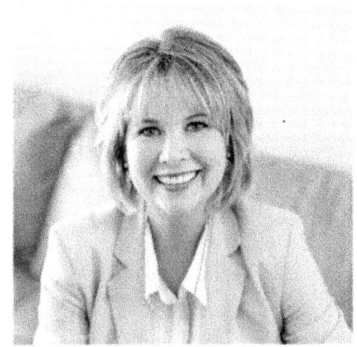

Guided by a family legacy of entrepreneurship, Michelle's journey is marked by a deep-rooted understanding of business dynamics and a relentless pursuit of personal growth. From her early years exploring her bustling 1970s neighborhood, where every day brought a new discovery, Michelle's insatiable curiosity set her on a path of lifelong learning. Mentored by her family's small businesses, she immersed herself in business studies and soon began a thriving career, rising through the ranks and building a stable, successful life.

Yet, despite her achievements, Michelle felt a profound pull toward something deeper. Realizing that the true heart of any business lay in its people, she shifted from business consulting to life coaching, finding her purpose in empowering women to break through personal and professional barriers. Today, Michelle combines her passion for growth and extensive business insights to inspire others, helping women uncover their potential and build lives and careers that resonate with meaning and purpose.

With her debut book, Michelle brings readers along on her journey, sharing the lessons, insights, and transformative moments that shaped her, offering a roadmap for anyone ready to pursue their own path to success.

For more information about the authors, speaking engagements, connecting with the authors, learning more about shifting your narrative, please visit our website at http://shiftingnarrativesbook.com/

www.ingramcontent.com/pod-product-compliance
Lightning Source LLC
Chambersburg PA
CBHW061700120626
46550CB00003B/1025